TALK WITH ME:
A STEP-BY-STEP CONVERSATION FRAMEWORK FOR TEACHING CONVERSATIONAL BALANCE AND FLUENCY FOR HIGH-FUNCTIONING INDIVIDUALS WITH AUTISM SPECTRUM DISORDERS

Kerry Mataya, M.S.Ed.
Ruth Aspy, Ph.D.
Hollis Shaffer

AN EVIDENCE-BASED STRATEGY

FUTURE HORIZONS

www.fhautism.com

info@fhautism.com

817.277.0727

©2017 Kerry Mataya, Ruth Aspy, Hollis Shaffer

All rights reserved. With the exception of the Appendix, no part of the material protected by this copyright notice may be reproduced or used in any form or by any means, electronic or mechanical, including photocopying, recording, or by any information storage and retrieval system, without the prior written permission of the copyright owner.

Publisher's Cataloging-in-Publication

Names:	Mataya, Kerry, author.	Aspy, Ruth, author.	Shaffer, Hollis, author.
Title:	Talk with me : a step-by-step conversation framework for teaching conversational balance and fluency : an evidence-based strategy / Kerry Mataya, Ruth Aspy, Hollis Shaffer.
	Authors have created a YouTube channel that contains a number of videos that show how to implement "Talk with Me". In addition, forms used in this curriculum are available for downloading.	Contents: Overview of the conversation framework -- Rules for implementing -- Embedded skills and related considerations -- The three steps -- Assessments -- Strategies for teaching -- Setting IEP goals -- References -- Appendices.	Includes bibliographical references.
Identifiers:	ISBN: 9781942197324	LCCN: 2017936814
Subjects:	LCSH: Autism spectrum disorders--Patients--Language.	Autism spectrum disorders--Patients--Means of communication.	Autism spectrum disorders--Patients--Life skills guides.	Autistic people--Language.	Autistic people--Means of communication.	Autistic people--Life skills guides.	Language disorders--Treatment.	Communicative competence--Study and teaching.	Conversation--Study and teaching.	Interpersonal communication--Study and teaching.	Discourse markers--Social aspects--Study and teaching.	Teachers of children with disabilities--Handbooks, manuals, etc.
Classification:	LCC: RC553.A88 M38 2017	DDC: 616.85/88206--dc23

TABLE OF CONTENTS

Introduction 1

Chapter 1: Overview of the Conversation Framework 5
    Why Is the Conversation Framework Needed? 5
        But Where to Start? 6
    What Is the Conversation Framework? 9
        The "Gestalt" of the Conversation Framework 9
            Step 1: Identify the Topic 11
            Step 2: Balance Asking Questions Within 0-2 Seconds 11
                      Balance Telling Stories Within 0-2 Seconds 11
                      Balance Making Comments Within 0-2 Seconds 11
            Step 3: Bridge the Topic 11

Chapter 2: Rules for Implementing the Conversation Framework 13
    Instructor Guidelines 13
    Explaining the Process and the "Why" 14
    Increasing Motivation 15
        Natural Environment Pictures 15
        Video Modeling 15
        Peer Feedback 15
        Teacher Feedback 16
        Assessment Scores 16
        "Try and See" and Evaluate 16
        Relationship Building 16
        Logical Reasoning 16
    Use of Categories 17
    Repeated Practice and Positive Experiences 17
    Group Placement 17
        Group Size 17
        Group Setting 18
        Group Participants 18
        Group Dynamics 18
    Gaining Administrator and Parent Support 25

Chapter 3: Embedded Skills and Related Considerations 27
    The Four Embedded Skills 27
        Active Listening 27
        Tone 28
        Timing 29
        Body Language 29
    The "Hidden Curriculum" 29
        Location 29
        Cultural Differences 30
        Relationships 30
            Role 30
            Age 30
            Closeness 30
        Gender 30
            Males in Conversation 31
            Females in Conversation 31
        Emotional Understanding 33

Chapter 4: The Three Steps of the Conversation Framework 35
    Step 1: Identify the Topic 35
        Common Challenges 35
        Identify the Overall Topic, Theme, or Subject of the Conversation 36
            General Topics 36
            Specific Topics 36
            Inferred Topics 36
        Identify the Weight of the Conversation 37
        Considerations 38
            Developmental Age 38
            Group Size and Setting 38
            Hesitation Time 38
            On- vs. Off-Topic 39
    Step 2: Balance Asking Questions, Telling Stories, and Making Comments
    Within 0-2 Seconds 39
        Common Challenges 39
        The Three Parts of Conversation 40
            Asking Questions 40
                Common Challenges 41
                Types of Questions 41
                      Questions to Start a Conversation 41
                      Follow-Up Questions 43
                      Reciprocal Questions 45
            Telling Stories 46
                Common Challenges 46
                Types of Stories 46
                      Sequential Stories 46
                      Informational Stories 47
                      Emotional Stories 47
                Reasons to Tell a Story 47
                      Stories to Start a Conversation 47
                      Related Stories 47
            Making Comments 48
                Common Challenges 48
                Types of Comments 49
                      Reflex Comments 49
                      Empathetic Comments 49
                      Response Comments 49
                      Satirical Comments 49
        Balancing the Conversation Using the Tally Mark Chart 49
            Balancing Conversation With Two People 50
            Balancing Conversation With a Small Group 50
            Balancing Conversation With a Large Group 51
        Considerations 54
            Age of Development 54
            Group Size and Setting 55
            Hesitation Time 55
    Step 3: Bridge the Topic 56
        Common Challenges 58
        Expanding the Topic 58
        Condensing the Topic 58
        Considerations 59
            Age of Development 59
            Group Size and Setting 59
            Hesitation Time 60

Chapter 5: Assessments for the Conversation Framework 61
- Measuring Ability and Progress 61
- Identifying the Topic 64
  - Assessment for Identifying the Topic (4 – 11 Years) 64
    - Part One 65
    - Part Two 67
    - Part Three 70
  - Assessment for Identifying the Topic (12 Years – Adult) 72
  - Assessment for Girl Conversation (12 Years – Adult) 79
  - Assessment for Implied Emotions (5 – 12 Years) 85
  - Assessment for Implied Emotions (12 Years – Adult) 87
  - Assessment for Inferred Meaning (12 Years – Adult) 90
  - Assessment for Recognizing Idioms and Sarcasm (7 Years – Adult) 93
- Balancing the Conversation 97
  - Assessment for Balancing Questions, Stories, and Comments 97
    - Tally Mark Chart (Two People) 97
- Asking Questions 97
  - Questions to Start a Conversation 97
    - Assessment for Starting a Conversation With School-Age People You Do Not Know 98
    - Assessment for Questions to Start a Conversation With Adults You Do Not Know 99
    - Assessment for Starting a Conversation With People You Know 99
  - Follow-Up Questions 101
    - Assessment for Follow-Up Questions – Prompted 101
    - Assessment for Follow-Up Questions – Unprompted 104
  - Reciprocal Questions 104
    - Assessment for Reciprocal Questions – Prompted 105
    - Assessment for Reciprocal Questions – Unprompted 105
- Telling Stories 106
  - Assessment for Sequential Stories 106
  - Assessment for Informational Stories 108
  - Assessment for Emotional Stories 110
  - Assessment for Related Stories 111
- Making Comments 113
  - Assessment for Empathetic Comments 113
  - Assessment for Response Comments 115
- Bridging the Topic 117
  - Assessment for Bridging the Topic 117

Chapter 6: Strategies for Teaching the Conversation Framework 119
- Methods for Teaching the Conversation Framework 121
- Required Tools 123
  - Conversation Topics List 123
  - Fast-Paced Audio Recordings 124
  - Tally Mark Chart 130
  - Bridge Visual 133
  - Common Category Chart 135
  - Transition Cards 137
- Drills 138
- Prompts 144
  - Verbal Prompts 144
  - Visual Prompts 147
  - Gesture Prompts 149
  - Behavior Prompts 149

Chapter 7: Setting IEP Goals Within the Conversation Framework 153
    IEP Goals for Step 1 153
    IEP Goals for Step 2 154
    IEP Goals for Step 3 156
    IEP Goals for Embedded Skills 157

References 159

Appendices 163
    A. Letter to Parent(s) 164
    B. Conversation Framework 166
    C. Conversation Topics List 167
    D. Conversation Topics List (With Pictures for Nonreaders) 168
    E. Topic 169
    F. General vs. Specific 170
    G. Weight 171
    H. Emotion List 172
    I. Timing 173
    J. Conversation vs. Whole-Group Listening 174
    K. Main Topic of Conversation 175
    L. Carrier Phrases for Asking Questions 176
    M. Carrier Phrases for Telling Stories 177
    N. Scripts for Comments 178
    O. Questions, Stories, Comments, Cheat Sheet 1 179
    P. Questions, Stories, Comments, Cheat Sheet 2 180
    Q. Bridge Visual 181
    R. Common Category Chart 182
    S. Transition Cards 183
    T. Data Collection Sheet, Q S C 186
    U. Data Collection Sheet, Bridging Topics 187
    V. Data Collection Sheet, Self-Report 188
    W. Guidelines for Balancing Conversation With
        Different Types of Participants 189
    X. Assessment for Balancing Questions, Stories, and Comments –
        Tally Mark Chart 192

Introduction

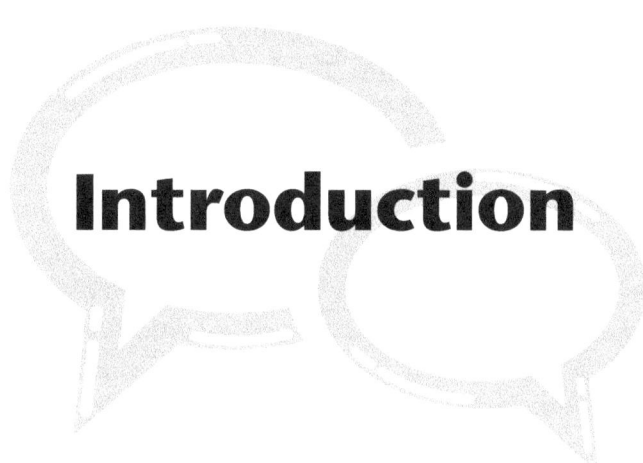

Conversation is everywhere – at the lunch table, at after-school activities, in the line for the water fountain, at overnight camp during downtime, at work with a coworker, or at a Thanksgiving gathering. Conversation requires effective communication and social interaction and is a requirement for developing or maintaining friendships. Conversation allows us to get information, give information, and to make others feel comfortable. Effective conversation skills may lead to successful relationships, independent living, and employment, whereas a lack of conversation skills may lead to failure in those areas.

Regardless of the setting, this critical skill – human conversation – is challenging for many individuals with high-functioning autism spectrum disorder (HF-ASD) – children and adults alike (Baron-Cohen, Wheelwright, Hill, Raste, & Plumb 2001; Stichter et al., 2010). Specifically, research has shown that individuals with ASD often have difficulty understanding context (Vermeulen, 2012) and process details in a conversation rather than seeing the overall conversational theme (Church et al., 2010; Scherf, Luna, Kimchi, Minshew, & Behrman, 2008). Difficulties with communication may lead to social isolation, social vulnerability, and sometimes bullying (Sofronoff, Dark, & Stone, 2011).

For these reasons, it is essential to equip individuals with ASD with effective conversational skills. Traditionally, the teaching of social skills, including conversation skills, friendship skills, and perspective-taking abilities, takes place in a group setting. Indeed, research has shown the benefits of group participation for learning these skills (MacKay, Knott, & Dunlop, 2007). However, it is often difficult to find a useful lesson that applies to everyone in a given group. As a result, leaders of social skills groups often find themselves picking and choosing lessons based on the needs of students in the group. That is, one lesson might apply to one person in the group, but not apply to the needs of others. Further, many social skills programs do not take place in real-life settings, making it difficult to apply newly learned skills in naturally occurring circumstances.

This is where the Conversation Framework comes in! This unique strategy provides an approach to assessing and teaching conversation skills in a group setting that is effective for most students who have difficulty engaging in conversations, including students with HF-ASD.

In use since 2005, the Conversation Framework has helped hundreds of individuals with HF-ASD learn how to have meaningful conversations. Parents who have used the conversation rules at home have reported an increase in conversation around the dinner table, including an awareness of asking follow-up questions about others' lives.

Teachers have reported success for their students, with greater acceptance from peers because of the increased reciprocal interactions with classmates. Teachers have also described an increase in listening skills, overall social awareness, and on-topic questions for students who have participated in groups using the Conversation Framework.

> *I'm excited about the changes I plan to make since being in Birmingham last week to learn the Conversation Framework. I hope that'll give me more of a vision of what I can do to reach more of the children and teens I teach. I'm also thinking I might try to start a group for the younger children (under 12), which I haven't done in the past. I decided to scratch the lesson that was planned for my teen group last night and just do a "conversation group" and learn about "questions, stories, and comments." I was dismayed to see that my teens couldn't carry on an on-topic conversation for more than 1½ minutes without becoming silent or making a drastic change in topic.*
>
> *They were interested in the change I made with the group and seemed excited to work on the new goals (although maybe a bit overwhelmed). One of them even said he couldn't believe that 50 minutes had already passed and we only have 10 minutes left. It's crazy to me that I had been following a curriculum, yet my teens were so unequipped. I look forward to seeing their progress because of what I learned from your group.*
>
> *– Social Group Leader, Alabama*

The Conversation Framework breaks down the elements of a conversation we must master in order to be proficient at carrying out a conversation. The framework was developed and refined across many years based on a review of the relevant research along with close observation of how people talk to each other – what conversations really sound like. Many find it difficult to teach conversation skills, but the Conversation Framework provides a simple and easy-to-implement process for teaching effective conversational habits.

The conversation rules presented in this book are specific enough to equip a high-functioning individual with ASD with the tools necessary to acquire conversation skills, and simple enough to be used at any age. The beauty of the Conversation Framework is that it does not change over time. That is, although kindergarteners may need to start at Step 1, whereas older students may be able to start at Step 2 or 3, the process of learning conversation is the same – the rules

> To help readers use this curriculum, we have created a YouTube channel, Talk with Me: Conversation Framework, that contains a number of videos that show how to implement the process at https://www.youtube.com/channel/UCUAFBVAd--StObl9n6OIh_A
>
> In addition, forms used in this curriculum are available for downloading at http://texasautism.com/blog/conversation-framework/
>
> Find Us On Instagram
> https://www.instagram.com/conversation_framework/?hl=en

that elementary school students learn are the same rules that they will need in adulthood. Learning these rules will help students be successful in conversation during the middle and high school years, when the hidden curriculum and use of slang become increasingly important, and during adulthood when mastery of conversation skills is necessary for participation in further education, employment, and the community.

INTRODUCTION

Specifically, research from the *National Autism Indicators Report: Transition into Young Adulthood* by Roux, Shattuck, Rast, Rava, and Kristy (2015) showed that the better the conversation skills an individual with ASD has, the less likely they are to be disconnected from society. Figure I.1 shows this relationship.

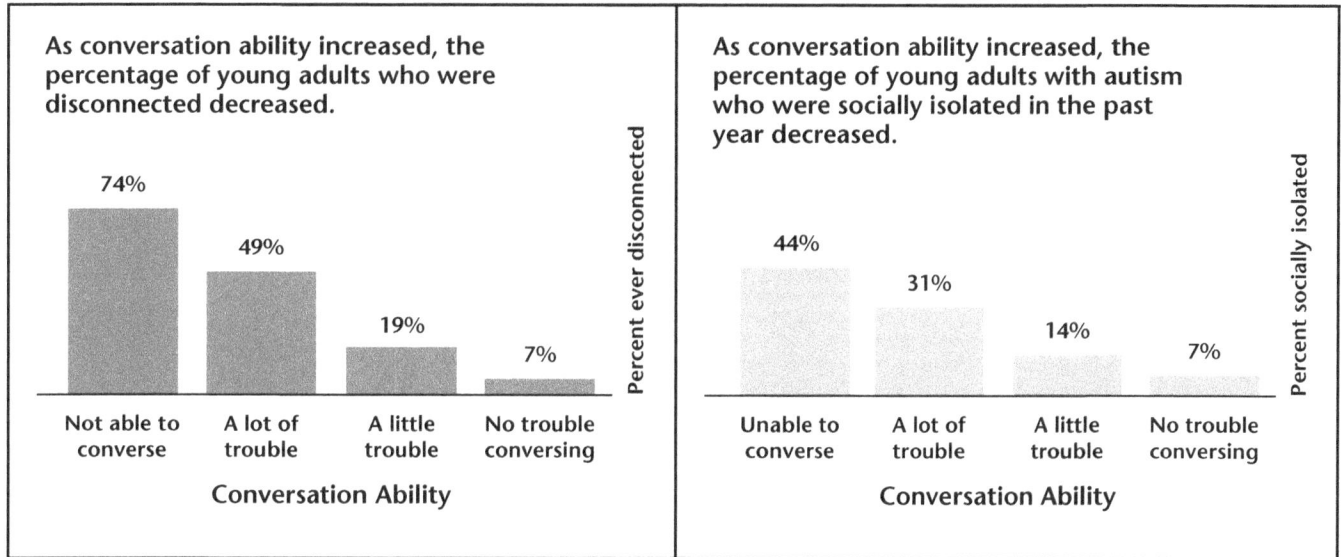

Figure I.1. Relationship between level of conversation skills and connection with society.
From Roux, A. M., Shattuck, P. T., Rast, J. E., Rava, J. A., & Anderson, K. A. (2015). *National autism indicators report: Transition into young adulthood* (p. 49). Philadelphia, PA: Life Course Outcomes Research Program, A.J. Drexel Autism Institute, Drexel University.

Similarly, employment is more likely for individuals with ASD in their 20s if they have conversation skills as shown below (Roux et al., 2015), as illustrated in Figure I.2.

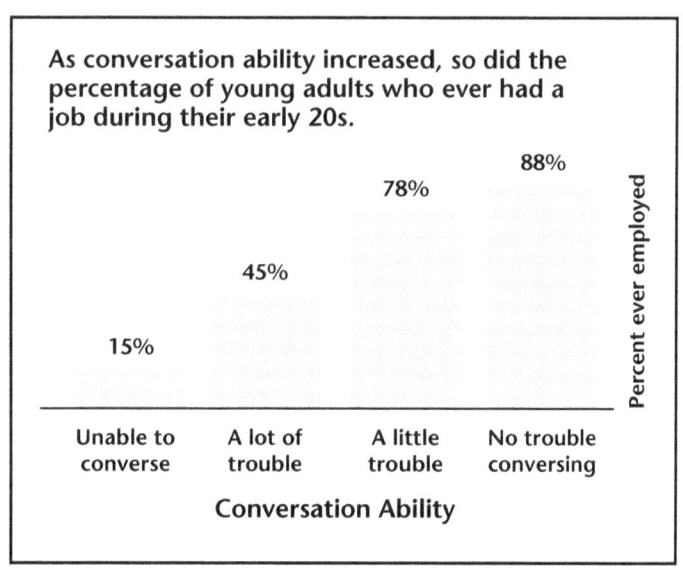

Figure I.2. Relationship between conversation skills and rate of employment.
From Roux, A. M., Shattuck, P. T., Rast, J. E., Rava, J. A., & Anderson, K. A. (2015). *National autism indicators report: Transition into young adulthood* (p. 58). Philadelphia, PA: Life Course Outcomes Research Program, A.J. Drexel Autism Institute, Drexel University.

> **Note**
>
> Several factors, including impaired language ability, history of bullying and teasing, anxiety, and difficulty participating in social situations, may impede an individual's success with the Conversation Framework. Although some of these issues will be improved through learning the Conversation Framework, other therapies or medical treatment may be necessary before the individual with ASD is able to fully benefit from the strategies used in the Conversation Framework approach.

CHAPTER 1
OVERVIEW OF THE CONVERSATION FRAMEWORK

Aside from basic greetings, goodbyes, and telephone etiquette, most conversation is unscripted. It is difficult to guess what people will be talking about, what they might ask, or where the conversation will go. This can make conversation challenging for everybody, but especially so for individuals with an autism spectrum disorder (ASD) who function best when the world around them, including the social world, is predictable (Aspy & Grossman, 2011). While numerous programs and curricula have been developed to address social skills deficits, including conversational skills, most are lacking for a number of reasons, including failure to address the complexity of conversations and taking into consideration the underlying characteristics of ASD.

WHY IS THE CONVERSATION FRAMEWORK NEEDED?

Table 1.1 lists behaviors that may indicate that someone has difficulty with conversation skills.

Table 1.1
Common Indicators of Deficits in Conversation Skills

• Brain "going blank," inability to think of anything to say	• Preference for conversation with someone not one's own age
• Inability to think of categories of conversation topics	• Failure to make comments in conversation
• Talking almost exclusively about self; one-sided conversations	• Failure to use nonverbal gestures to show interest in conversation
• Failure to ask questions about others	• Lack of awareness that others may not be interested in what is being said
• Asking too many questions	• Often feeling cut off or interrupted
• Asking questions even when already knowing the answer	• Often interrupting others
• Not wanting to listen or join conversations of non-interest	• Difficulty with timing in conversation
• Telling longwinded stories	• Talking too loudly or too quietly
• Difficulty telling relevant or key details of a story	• Anxiety about talking to new people
• Starting at the beginning of a story and including every detail	• Anxiety about talking to someone of the opposite gender
• Giving one-word answers in response to a question	• Anxiety about talking in large groups
• Difficulty developing social reciprocity	• Anxiety about not knowing what to say
• Waiting for others to initiate conversation	• Fear of saying something wrong
• Requiring others to keep the conversation going	

Learning to carry on a successful conversation requires a lot of practice for students with high-functioning ASD (HF-ASD). Knowing this, it is important to start teaching and practicing as soon as it is clear that a student has a deficit in conversation (see also Chapter 5 on assessment).

But Where to Start?

Many professionals, including speech-language pathologists (SLPs), psychologists, counselors, special education teachers, autism specialists, and classroom teachers, teach conversation skills, often with the use of peer helpers. Aspects of conversation addressed through typical strategies generally include the following:

- Eye contact
- Equal turns
- Greeting others
- Starting a conversation
- Maintaining a conversation
- Ending a conversation
- Joining a conversation
- Showing interest
- Listening carefully
- Making the other person feel comfortable
- Allowing the other person time to think or speak

The problem with teaching conversation using this approach is that the rules for conversation are malleable and changing. Conversations do not always begin with a greeting. Good conversations do not always have an equal number of exchanges. And the nature of a conversation changes depending on characteristics of the conversation partners such as familiarity, age, and gender.

Further, if conversation skills are included in a student's individualized education program (IEP), the objectives are often written for a specific number of exchanges or a specific length of time (e.g., hold a 3-minute conversation with four exchanges). Although this is well intended, a student may master these objectives and still not be able to participate in a conversation in a socially functional way. Does an IEP objective to have a 3-minute conversation indicate which conversation skill is deficient? Does the number of minutes that a conversation lasts indicate the quality of the conversation? If the objective is written for five exchanges in a conversation, how long is the student really able to maintain a conversation? Is a higher number of exchanges necessarily an improvement? Would the family know how to generalize this skill to the home environment?

Another reason why many standard social skills programs are not effective is that difficulties with conversation are often considered to be caused by social skills deficits; however, in reality, they may also be related to deficits in executive functioning and underlying cognition challenges often present in those with HF-ASD, as described in Table 1.2. Thus, difficulty with organizing and processing social information can make conversation challenging. Therefore, strategies to improve conversation skills must address this broad range of interrelated underlying needs – social and cognitive.

CHAPTER 1: OVERVIEW OF THE CONVERSATION FRAMEWORK

Table 1.2
Common Deficits in Executive Functioning and Cognition of Individuals With HF-ASD

Area of Cognitive Functioning	Support in Literature and Research
Processing Speed	Individuals with ASD have "restrained" processing. That is, they process information at a slower pace than typically developing peers (Williams et al., 2013).
Central Coherence	According to Vermeulen (2012), individuals with HF-ASD often have difficulty in using context to determine if someone already knows something or if a fact is obvious before they share information. As a result, they often elaborate on irrelevant details, not understanding which information is important and which is not. Individuals with HF-ASD also interpret and form categories differently than others, with specific attention to detail rather than big picture thinking (Church et al., 2010; Scherf et al., 2009).
Theory of Mind	Flood, Hare, and Wallis (2011) found that individuals with HF-ASD demonstrated deficits with regard to attributing intentions. Individuals with ASD often have difficulty recognizing emotions or perceptions of others (Stichter et al., 2010). Individuals with HF-ASD express decreased emotional responses to situations compared to neurotypical controls (Kleinhans et al., 2010).
Flexibility	Difficulty with thinking flexibly is a diagnostic characteristic of ASD (American Psychiatric Association [APA], 2013).
Attending	A high percentage of individuals with ASD exhibit symptoms of an attention deficit disorder (Volkmar et al., 2014). Individuals with ASD may be successful in attending to topics of high interest but with little attention to topics of low interest (Gagnon & Myles, 2016; Tanidir & Mukaddes, 2014).
Nonverbal Communication	Social skills deficits may include deficits in interpreting gestures and difficulty with face recognition (Wilson, Brock, & Palermo, 2010).
Memory (Rote and Meaningful)	Deficits in auditory and visual memory have been found to increase with the complexity of the material presented (Williams, Goldstein, & Minshew, 2006). Researchers noted deficits in auditory working memory in individuals with ASD (Holdnack, Goldstein, & Drozdick, 2011).
Joint Attention	Joint attention means actively sharing attention. It is the basis for shared understanding and communication. Deficits in joint attention among individuals with ASD are well established in the research (Ames & Fletcher-Watson, 2010).

The following describes a student, Carrie, who had difficulty maintaining a reciprocal conversation, despite years of traditional social skills training. This young woman was diagnosed with Asperger Syndrome (now diagnosed as ASD; APA, 2013) in middle school and received accommodations and basic social skill services throughout her middle and high school years.

Carrie was a sophomore at a small private college when she sought help. She had concerns about a lack of friendships. When she was in high school, she was involved in band and had a core group of male and female students that she was around on a daily basis. At that time, she felt social connections regardless of her failure to initiate interactions. She described being around others and feeling part of a group. After her first year of college, she described feeling lonely and realized that she had difficulty maintaining relationships with others.

When Carrie came in for her first session, she waited for the examiner to initiate conversation. She was able to answer questions and told multiple stories about her own life. Her conversation was pleasant, but it was one-sided – focused on herself and her experiences. She did not ask questions to start a conversation or follow-up questions about the examiner. She was not connecting with others' lives and experiences because she did not know how to show interest through asking questions about another person. When prompted to ask a question of the examiner, she was quiet and looked like she was thinking. When given additional time to come up with a question, she eventually said, "I don't know." When given even more time, she said, "I can't think of anything."

As is true for many with ASD, Carrie needed a framework to learn how to participate successfully in a conversation. She needed to know what to say and how to retrieve that information. Giving additional processing time to come up with something to say was not effective for her. In fact, the more she thought about what she did not know how to say, the more her anxiety increased. As with many individuals with ASD, her anxiety impaired her conversation performance.

Indeed, because many individuals with HF-ASD demonstrate high levels of anxiety (Hare, Wood, Wastell, & Skirrow, 2014), one goal of the Conversation Framework is to use repetition and skill development to decrease anxiety in everyday conversations. Rather than verbalizing "I don't know what to say" or "My mind blanked out," or quietly staring, individuals are able to initiate or contribute to a conversation on topic using the parts of conversation outlined in the Conversation Framework.

Negative Effects of Anxiety
- Anxiety increases "blanking out"
- Anxiety decreases confidence
- Anxiety decreases eye contact
- Anxiety increases with lack of predictability
- Anxiety increases when over-prompted or given too many directions:
  – "Sit up"
  – "Make good eye contact"
  – "Lean forward"
  – "Listen"
  – "Nod your head"
  – "Ask questions"

CHAPTER 1: OVERVIEW OF THE CONVERSATION FRAMEWORK

The shortcomings of traditional approaches to teaching conversation skills outlined above prompted the development of the Conversation Framework, which takes all of these areas into account and results in enabling individuals with HF-ASD to have effective conversations.

WHAT IS THE CONVERSATION FRAMEWORK?

Conversation can be complex, making it difficult to break down its components to comprehensively and systematically teach the rules, as we do when teaching many other skills. The Conversation Framework is a comprehensive step-by-step process designed to teach teachers, parents, SLPs, and others how to help high-functioning students with ASD to engage in effective conversation with others. It is an instructional tool that facilitates understanding of conversation by providing the gestalt, or "big picture," of how to teach conversation.

The overall goal of the Conversation Framework is to provide concrete steps for teaching conversation that promote retention of skills and natural conversation in a wide range of settings with a variety of people. Through use of the Conversation Framework, specific areas within a conversation are targeted and replacement conversation skills are taught that assist with behavior, awareness, and perspective taking.

Reaching Goals

Many years ago I sat in a team meeting discussing the lack of conversation skills for a high-functioning kindergarten student with ASD. The IEP team was concerned about his one-sided talking "at" others and his disruption of the class when he interrupted the teacher to make irrelevant comments during whole-group instruction. I suggested adding IEP benchmarks for specific areas of conversation, including knowing the topic, asking questions, telling stories, and making comments. An autism advocate at the meeting responded that the child was years away from learning these skills and concluded that it would be several years before he would be able to ask a follow up question. She suggested benchmarks for walking independently in the hallway. However, through use of the Conversation Framework, eight months later the student often knew the topic and asked independent follow-up questions, as evidenced through teacher observation and data collection. After learning the Conversation Framework, his off-topic comments decreased, on topic comments increased, and raising his hand and awareness of others increased. His overall behavior significantly improved.

– Kerry Mataya

The "Gestalt" of the Conversation Framework

Wing (1981) described the typical conversation style of somebody with ASD as "one-sided." For that reason, a major step of the Conversation Framework focuses on how to "balance" rather than monopolize the conversation, by helping students visualize the entire framework. The word *visualize* is significant here. Most people with ASD – but not all – process information more effectively when it is presented visually rather than relying only on auditory input. (Previous cognitive assessments that may have been completed are a good resource if you are unsure of somebody's learning style.)

Despite focusing on the big picture, the Conversation Framework is taught one step at a time. Because high-functioning individuals with ASD often have difficulty multitasking, the Conversation Framework allows the student to learn skills step-by-step. That is one step must be mastered and become consistent across settings before the next step is introduced. To that end, the Conversation Framework uses repetition and best practice techniques that allow skills to become habitual. Indeed, because real conversation tends to move rapidly, some skills in the framework are not considered to be mastered until they are routinely exhibited within 0 to 2 seconds. This will be discussed more fully in later chapters. Figure 1.1 illustrates the gestalt ("big picture") of the Conversation Framework.

CONVERSATION STEPS	
STEP 1: Identify the Topic	Embedded Skills: Listening, Tone, Timing, Body Language
Topic _____	
STEP 2: Balance – Asking Questions, Telling Stories, and Making Comments Within 0-2 Seconds	
Q Asking Questions	
S Telling Stories	
C Making Comments	
STEP 3: Bridge the Topic	

Figure 1.1. Overview of the steps of the Conversation Framework.

CHAPTER 1: OVERVIEW OF THE CONVERSATION FRAMEWORK

As outlined in Figure 1.1, and described in more detail below, the Conversation Framework consists of three steps: (a) identifying the topic; (b) balancing asking questions, telling stories, and making comments within 0-2 seconds; and (c) bridging the topic. Although not the main focus, listening, tone, timing, and body language are embedded into each of the steps.

Let's look briefly at each step within the Conversation Framework. Additional information on each step is provided in Chapters 4, 5, and 6.

Step 1 – Identify the Topic

Knowing the topic is the first step toward having an effective conversation. To identify the topic, you must be able to identify the subject of a conversation, the weight or seriousness of what is being discussed, the implied emotion within the conversation, and the inferred meaning of the conversation. The concept of "on topic" vs. "off topic" is also addressed.

Step 2 – Balancing Asking Questions, Telling Stories, and Making Comments Within 0-2 Seconds

The term *balance* is used here to refer to creating an equal distribution of questions, stories, and comments both with regard to one's own utterances and in proportion to others' statements.

- **Balancing Asking Questions Within 0-2 Seconds**
  Asking questions is essential to keeping a conversation going. There are three different types of questions: (a) questions to start a conversation, (b) follow-up questions about what someone just said, and (c) reciprocal questions. Asking questions allows you to find out information from others, as well as let someone know you are interested in what they have to say. In general, people like to talk about themselves and their experiences. There are times we may not be interested in what someone has to say, but we ask a question anyway because it shows interest in others.

- **Balancing Telling Stories Within 0-2 Seconds**
  Telling stories is a significant component of having a conversation. Conversations without stories are boring. Stories can be based on sequential, informational, or emotional events. There are two different types of stories: (a) stories to start a conversation and (b) related stories. Stories allow you to give information in a logical format. They vary in length.

- **Balancing Making Comments Within 0-2 Seconds**
  Making relevant comments is an important part of mastering conversation. Making comments allows you to show interest in what others are saying and makes others feel comfortable. There are four types of comments: (a) reflex comments, (b) empathetic comments, (c) response comments, and (d) sarcastic comments.

Step 3 – Bridge the Topic

Bridging the topic is the most vital skill for maintaining a longer conversation. Once the other areas of the Conversation Framework are mastered, the next step is learning to bridge from one topic to a related topic without appearing to make a drastic change in the conversation. There are three types of bridging topics: (a) expanding categories, (b) condensing categories, and (c) smooth transitions.

It is important to show fluency within each step of the Conversation Framework to be proficient in natural conversations.

CHAPTER 2
RULES FOR IMPLEMENTING THE CONVERSATION FRAMEWORK

Before utilizing the Conversation Framework, it is important to recognize and accept that the individual components are most effective when used in the specific order outlined in this book.

INSTRUCTOR GUIDELINES

1. Become totally comfortable using the Conversation Framework; however, know that being familiar with the process is not enough. Anyone implementing the Conversation Framework should know the individual steps and the sequential order utilized throughout this book. For successful implementation of the Conversation Framework, implementers should also use the vocabulary and skills associated with each step.

2. Carefully review assessment results (see Chapter 5) to determine a starting point for each student learning the Conversation Framework.

3. To ensure mastery of the Conversation Framework, both individual and group sessions are essential. Individual services alone will not bring about conversation fluency without opportunities to generalize the skills in a group setting, nor will a group setting bring about conversation fluency without the student's individual needs being addressed. Too often a student's needs get overlooked in a group setting. Likewise, a student's skills may not generalize from an individual setting to a group setting because the student has not properly practiced timing and initiation with enough repeated practice to combat the increased anxiety that comes from having conversation with a group of peers. Please refer to pages 17-19 and Chapter 4 for more information on group placement.

4. Collect and review data on a regular basis to monitor progress. The data provide a basis for determining if there is a need to reset goals or to adjust the setting for working through the Conversation Framework. Please refer to Chapter 5 for more information on data collection. Regardless of the type of data collection that is chosen, it should be meaningful and should be used to track progress over time. Individualize the data collection to the needs of the student. Options and ideas for data collection may be found in Appendices T, U, and V.

With these basic guidelines in mind, we will now look at other elements necessary for ensuring successful implementation of the Conversation Framework.

EXPLAINING THE PROCESS AND THE "WHY"

It is important to explain the overall Conversation Framework to the person with autism spectrum disorder (ASD) at the very beginning. This explanation, stressing the importance of knowing the framework, is simple and straightforward. Students' motivation to learn the framework typically improves when they feel encouraged, recognize why conversation skills are needed, and understand that the skills are attainable.

How the Conversation Framework is presented or packaged affects students' motivation to learn it. Individualize the "why" for each student. If your student is uninterested in learning conversation, then directly describe the importance of conversation; for example, "This is what people do, and it's expected in our society." Some students have to experience success before they will buy into the process. Remember to encourage your students by reminding them that they can do it and that they will be able to learn the skills. Validate their feelings if you know that it is hard for them. Be mindful that some students do not register an awkward pause or become uncomfortable during conversation. This should be factored in when determining a person's motivation. For more information on teaching the Conversation Framework, please refer to Chapter 6.

Here are some examples of explaining the process:

- "Conversation is only asking questions, telling stories, and making comments."
- "You have to do one of those three things to be in the conversation."
- "I'll help you get good at all of those parts of conversation."
- "Being good at all of those parts of conversation will help you be able to talk to anyone anywhere."
- "We'll just work on it until you get it."
- "I'll teach you how to listen for a pause to jump in."
- "We won't move on to the next step until you've mastered the first step."
- "Practicing will help you to be more comfortable."
- "This is something that will help you later in life."
- "Do you want to feel more comfortable in conversation?"
- "You may not feel uncomfortable with awkward silence, but other people do. It's important for everyone to feel comfortable in the conversation, otherwise people do not continue the conversation."
- "You may be saying that you do not like people or conversation. You may have had bad experiences in the past. I'm here to help you to be more successful. I want conversation to work for you. Even if you don't want friends right now, I want you to teach you to have conversation in case you want friends at some point in your life."
- "Conversation allows you to get information, give information, and make others feel comfortable."

CHAPTER 2: RULES FOR IMPLEMENTING THE CONVERSATION FRAMEWORK

> **Student Ability**
>
> The Conversation Framework addresses conversation skills for students with average to above-average language skills. If you have concerns about your student's use of syntax (sentence patterns, phrase elaboration, verb phrase) or semantics (meaning), please consult with a professional such as a speech-language pathologist (SLP). Students with below-average expressive language skills can benefit from the program; however, progress may be slower.

INCREASING MOTIVATION

Getting a student's buy-in is essential to increasing overall motivation for learning a new or difficult skill.

Steps for getting the student's buy-in to work on something include:
1. Student has to agree that what he/she is doing is a problem.
2. Student has to understand why it is a problem.
3. Student has to have opportunities to practice replacement skills and experience success.
4. Student has to master replacement skills.

Once students have mastered a new skill, they are more motivated to take on another challenge. In short, success gains momentum.

The following are some specific strategies for gaining a student's buy-in:

Natural Environment Pictures
Take pictures of times when the student is doing things differently than others. Use the pictures as a teaching tool for self-awareness or perspective taking. For example, photos can be useful for recognizing body language showing a peer's disinterest as well as teaching body language to make conversation believable.

Video Modeling
Similarly, take videos of times when the student is doing things that are different than others. Use the videos as a teaching tool for self-awareness or perspective taking. For example, video modeling can be useful for teaching the content of any part of the Conversation Framework steps.

Peer Feedback
Ask a peer(s) to talk to the student about his strengths and challenges in order to show the student that you are not the only one who thinks he is doing something different than others. Be prepared that the student may make comments (e.g., "You're making him say that") accusing you of coercing the peer into making comments that he or she does not believe. Such comments may signal a deficit in theory of mind (ToM) – the ability to recognize and attribute mental states not only in onself but

in others, and to understand that feelings and beliefs we have may be different than others – and make this strategy ineffective unless the student knew that the peer was approaching him on his or her own.

Teacher Feedback

Ask a teacher(s) to talk to the student to give the student specific feedback on strengths and challenges. Sometimes awareness is all that is needed to create motivation and buy-in. This strategy is typically most effective if a student has a positive relationship and trust with the teacher providing the feedback.

Assessment Scores

If standardized assessments are available and relevant, review the assessment(s) with the student to objectively show a skill deficit in a specific area (e.g., processing speed on WISC-5). Assessments may be formal or informal. For the purposes of showing conversation deficits, the assessments in Chapter 5 will provide sufficient information to understand the strengths and challenges that your student is experiencing.

"Try and See" and Evaluate

Many times adults are quick to dismiss students' ideas – especially students with high-functioning ASD (HF-ASD). It can create a positive relationship if a student is validated or the adult agrees to try his idea first on a time-limited basis (e.g., "We will try your idea and evaluate it in two weeks). Although this strategy is not acceptable for all skills, it is appropriate in some instances when a student is working on his conversation deficits.

Relationship Building

If you have a positive relationship with your student, use this relationship to convince her to try something (e.g., "How many times have I been wrong about you?"). Students who have had negative experiences in the past may use avoidance tactics as a way to escape learning the skills involved in the Conversation Framework. Positive relationships can often motivate a student to try again, even if prior efforts were unsuccessful.

Logical Reasoning

Use of logical reasoning can be very effective for many students with HF-ASD. That is, logically show the student how what he is doing may negatively impact him – whether it prevents him from eventually getting what he wants or why it is harmful to the situation or person (e.g., "When you do this, people leave; "If this happens, it will be difficult to get into that college.").

USE OF CATEGORIES

The Conversation Framework breaks conversation into categories. Categories teach how to interpret information and group like pieces of information together, while helping students with HF-ASD to interpret and participate in conversation. High-functioning individuals with ASD often interpret and form categories differently than others. For example, they may tend to pay specific attention to detail rather than to focus on the big picture (Church et al., 2010; Scherf et al., 2009). While attention to detail can be helpful for many life tasks, attending to minute details within a story tends to negatively impact fluent conversation with others. Focused on teaching categories, Bock (1994, 1999) found that children with ASD achieved generalization and maintenance through interventions using categorical thinking. The use of categories is woven throughout the Conversation Framework.

REPEATED PRACTICE AND POSITIVE EXPERIENCES

Effective use of the Conversation Framework rests on repeated practice and positive experiences. To change conversational habits, opportunities for repeated practice and positive experiences are mandatory. We are all more likely to try out a skill in a new setting if we have previously experienced success.

GROUP PLACEMENT

Organizations such as clinics or public and private schools that serve those with ASD often provide some services in group settings. Group sessions provide a built-in opportunity for generalization. In other words, rather than interacting with just one person, the participants in the group have the opportunity to practice their new skills with others in the group as well. Group sessions also provide more opportunities to learn about a range of social interactions and challenges.

For these same reasons, the Conversation Framework is most often taught in group sessions; however, not everyone who is learning the Conversation Framework will be ready for a group. Factors that may impact readiness to participate in a group include sensory needs, anxiety, and severe disruptive behaviors. However, the presence of these challenges does not necessarily prohibit a student from being in a group setting if the right supports are present. When a participant is ready for groups, multiple prerequisites are required.

Most fundamentally, it is important for students to feel comfortable in a conversation group. The main goal of group placements is to create a safe environment where all students are able to learn and practice based on their individual progress with the Conversation Framework. Four key factors with regard to placement affect the outcome of students' conversation development: group size, group setting, group participants, and group dynamics.

Group Size

Some individuals need individual sessions with an adult or a small group in the beginning, whereas others learn more quickly in a medium or large group. The group size should be individualized based on the needs of each participant. Further guidelines for determining group size are discussed in Chapter 4.

> **Group Sizes**
> - Individual session with adult
> - Small group – 1 to 4 peers
> - Medium group – 5 to 7 peers
> - Large group – 8+ peers

Group Setting

With regard to setting, noises can be particularly distracting to individuals with HF-ASD. Try to minimize background noise as much as possible, especially for students who are new to participating in a conversation group. Also, certain types of lighting and sounds may be painful to students with ASD because of their sensory issues. These vary from person to person, so consult with an occupational therapist (OT) with training and experience in addressing sensory differences, as needed.

Conversations take place in a wide range of settings; therefore, the eventual goal is for a student to be able to participate in conversations under a range of conditions. These include the following:

- Without background noise
- With background noise (constant)
- With background noise (changing)
- Unstructured setting (hallway transition, recess, lunch)
- Structured setting (classroom)

Sitting and Standing

Whether we sit or stand while engaged in a conversation is controlled by the setting and affect the dynamics of a group, so be sure to practice conversation both while standing and sitting.

Group Participants

When putting together a group to practice conversation, it is essential to consider the types of people within the group. For example, a person who is constantly telling long-winded stories is a "bad fit" for somebody who talks very little because there will be very few pauses to say something. In addition, the person who tells a lot of stories will talk more than usual to compensate for the person who is saying very little.

Many group leaders want to put all students with ASD in the same social skills group. This is not always a good idea, however, as it may result in a lack of progress because of the mismatch of expressive language patterns. Nevertheless, there may be times when you do not have the luxury to choose who is in a group. If this is the case, even if not ideal, it is still possible to teach to each person's individual needs.

Group Dynamics

Group dynamics refer to interactions between group participants – the flow of the conversation created by the participants. A welcoming environment where students can learn and make mistakes fosters positive group dynamics.

If a group participant talks very little, this may cause someone else to talk a lot more than they would in another situation. When working with a small social group, you will likely have one student who is working on learning the topic. It is not fair to put someone in a conversation in which they have no idea what is being discussed. Therefore, it is imperative to figure out *if* a student knows the topic ahead of time; for example, by asking the student privately if he is OK with you asking him what the topic is in the middle of the group. If he is not, you may need to use fast-paced audio recordings (see

CHAPTER 2: RULES FOR IMPLEMENTING THE CONVERSATION FRAMEWORK

pages 124-129) to determine if he is able to identify the topic. If possible, it is better to record the conversation he is in and ask him about the topic privately.

Ultimately, you may not know which group dynamic will work best with a particular student until you try out different group settings to find out which group dynamic is the best fit for each student.

Positive behavior is a critical component of an effective conversation group, whereas negative behavior can have a very damaging effect. Unfortunately, many adults trained in teaching conversation skills are not effectively trained in how to deal with behavioral concerns such as a sensitive student crying whenever the group talks about M-rated (mature) video games or a student becoming frustrated when he is interrupted. To compensate for difficulties with addressing challenging behaviors, many adults structure conversation groups by overfocusing on turn taking or specific topic maintenance, which does not replicate real-life conversation. The book *High-Functioning Autism and Difficult Moments* (Myles & Aspy, 2016) provides strategies for understanding and addressing behavioral concerns while keeping a focus on the underlying needs associated with ASD. Knowing how to effectively address behavioral challenges will allow the adult the opportunity to focus her attention on teaching the steps within the Conversation Framework.

Conversation Example With Prompts

The following example shows how prompts are used within a natural conversation. Throughout our sessions, we use a combination of verbal and visual prompts. The prompts are used to guide, redirect, refocus, and encourage our students.

Age: 13 – 19 years old

Gender: Male

Group Size: 8 students

Conversational Goals:

    Amar – Step 3: Bridging the Topic

    Richard – Step 2: Balancing the Conversation (Including Initiation or Jumping Into the Conversation With a Question, Story, or Comment)

    Walsh – Step 2: Balancing the Conversation (Including Asking Questions About Others)

    Andrew – Step 2: Balancing the Conversation (Including Asking Questions About Others)

    Will – Step 2: Balancing the Conversation (Including Staying on Topic Without Changing It to His Special Interest)

    Henry – Step 2: Balancing the Conversation (On Topics of Non-Interest)

    Christian – Step 2: Balancing the Conversation (Including Initiation or Jumping Into the Conversation With a Question, Story, or Comment)

    Taylor – Step 2: Balancing the Conversation (On Topics of Non-Interest)

Strategy for Teaching the Conversation Framework

    Natural Conversation

TALK WITH ME

Student's Conversation	Adult Prompts
Amar: Speaking of Teenage Mutant Ninja Turtles, what is your favorite Teenage Mutant Ninja Turtle?	
	Mrs. Kerry: We weren't speaking of Teenage Mutant Ninja Turtles. What is Teenage Mutant Ninja Turtles?
Richard: Cartoon. Walsh: Movie.	
	Mrs. Kerry: (*handed out Conversation Topics visual support*) It can be a movie or whatever but you've got to bridge it from school. You would have to say speaking of things we do or speaking of places we go. You would have to bridge it from school. Do you want to try one more time?
Amar: Speaking about going places …	
	Mrs. Kerry: That reminds me of …
Amar: Going to the movies like the last time I had seen the movie *Teenage Mutant Ninja Turtles*.	
	Mrs. Kerry: So say the whole thing. Speaking of going places, that reminds me of …
Amar: Speaking of going places, that reminds me of going to the movies when I saw the movie *Teenage Mutant Ninja Turtles*.	
	Mrs. Kerry: And then?
Amar: Does anybody else like Teenage Mutant Ninja Turtles? Andrew: No, just no. Walsh and Richard: I do. Amar: Why don't you like Teenage Mutant Ninja Turtles? Walsh: Yeah, why you be hating on Teenage Mutant Ninja Turtles? Richard: it's a great cartoon. Especially the old one. Andrew: The original cartoon, that was good I liked the original cartoon, but now I don't. Walsh: The new one is like "eh." Walsh, Richard, Andrew, Amar: Yeah. Andrew: The 2003 series was awesome, but the way it is now, it sucks.	

CHAPTER 2: RULES FOR IMPLEMENTING THE CONVERSATION FRAMEWORK

Student's Conversation	Adult Prompts
Will: I just want to know when Hollis is getting back with pizza.	
	Mrs. Kerry: It's off topic and you're going to have to compartmentalize that and think about this. Christian, jump in. What are they talking about?
Christian: Teenage Mutant Ninja Turtles.	
	Mrs. Kerry: You can like the topic or not like it, but jump in and tell a story. Your story can even be that you don't like it.
Christian: What's the movie about? Walsh: Which one? Christian: The new one. Taylor: I'm not sure what to think about that one. Richard: There are a few live-action *Teenage Mutant Ninja Turtles* movies, but I never really saw the new ones, but I have the three old ones. Amar: Did you like Shredder? Walsh: He was cool. In the new cartoons, they just added so many new villains, and it's hard to keep track of them.	
	Mrs. Kerry: OK, jump in on topic, Henry.
Henry: Really, all I truly know about TMNT … I don't really know too much about it. I've only watched a couple movies. There's four turtles and a samurai. Amar: That's the Shredder. Andrew: We've already established that, Amar.	
	Mrs. Kerry: Bridge it to something else then instead of calling people out.
Andrew: I was about to! Amar: Andrew, that's mean. Don't stare at me.	
	Mrs. Kerry: OK, I need you to stop, Amar. Bridge it to something else, Andrew.
Andrew: Teenage Mutant Ninja Turtles was only just a comic. They were produced by Marvel.	
	Mrs. Kerry: Speaking of …

TALK WITH ME

Student's Conversation	Adult Prompts
Andrew: Speaking of major things that were produced by Marvel, when do you think they're gonna come out with that third *GI Joe* movie?	
Henry: GI Joe started in Marvel?	
Andrew: Yes, it did. So did Transformers, Amar.	
Henry: You mean the comics?	
Andrew: Yes, that's what started it all.	
Amar: Yes, I am ready for *Transformers Part Five*.	
Andrew: I'm just waiting for *GI Joe 3*. Duke lives.	
Walsh: I'm a little confused. Marvel ran the comics of Teenage Mutant Ninja Turtles. So Disney owns Marvel, so then why …?	
Andrew: No they don't. They only own enough shares in the company to be able to produce the movies and stuff without permission because they own enough stock. They don't own the entire company. They just own a large percentage of it.	
Walsh: So they own the right to make TV shows?	
Andrew: Yes, they have enough stock for the rights.	
Walsh: So then, wouldn't that mean that Nickelodeon would have to cancel their TV show because technically Disney should own the rights?	
Andrew: Well, Teenage Mutant Ninja Turtles and GI Joe got so big that they separated from Marvel a while ago. They just became an independent story line.	
Walsh: That makes sense. Speaking of Disney owning stuff, who was upset by Disney buying Star Wars?	
Andrew: Well frankly, with Star Wars Rebels, I'm actually surprised by how good they've done.	
Walsh: Well see, I loved the original cartoon series that ran on cartoon network.	
Henry: Clone Wars?	
Walsh: Yeah because it actually continued the first three episodes. I'm more interested in what happened in those than in the Rebels.	
Andrew: But Rebels is frankly better than I thought it would be, so I'm actually excited to see what they do with this new movie.	
Taylor: Speaking of, I actually went to Disney over the weekend.	
Andrew: Oh, you mean with the Star Wars simulator ride where they pick a spy?	
Taylor: Yeah, that actually happened to me the first time I rode it.	
Andrew: And you were the spy?	
Taylor: Yes, they picked me.	
Andrew: I wanted to be the spy, so I rode it over and over again.	
Taylor: And you weren't picked?	
Andrew: No, but I did get to make a double-bladed light saber with a purple blade and those cool wrist guards that Count Dooku has.	
	Mrs. Kerry: What's the topic, Will?
Will: Star Wars.	

CHAPTER 2: RULES FOR IMPLEMENTING THE CONVERSATION FRAMEWORK

Student's Conversation	Adult Prompts
	Mrs. Kerry: And it moved on to …?
Will: Disney.	
	Mrs. Kerry: OK. Jump in.
Amar: I have not watched *Star Wars* in a very long time, but I thought it was OK though. Andrew: OK? Have you been listening? We've been talking about how awesome it is, and you're like, "Oh, it's OK." Amar: I don't hate it. Why would you think I hate it? Andrew: I never said that I think you hate it. I just think that the other people who have talked about Star Wars were like, "Oh, yeah it's great," and you were like, "It's OK." Amar: Well I would just like to say that I might see the new Star Wars movie coming out. Walsh: I didn't even see the trailer. I am not seeing a single thing because I don't want to see it. Henry: What is the new Star Wars gonna be called anyway? Andrew: I'm not sure, but I … Walsh: *Star Wars 7. Star Wars* episode 7 or whatever.	
	Mrs. Kerry: Hold on. Topic? (*Pointing to Christian*)
Christian: *Star Wars.*	
	Mrs. Kerry: OK. Jump in.
Henry: So the name is …? Andrew: We don't know. They haven't told us yet. But um, it's gonna be like when Luke is …	
	Mrs. Kerry: Shhh.
Christian: What are y'all talking about? Walsh: You (Mrs. Kerry) want me to tell him what we're talking about?	
	Mrs. Kerry: Yeah.
Walsh: We're talking about Star Wars and the TV shows and movie that are coming out this year. Taylor: And Disney. Andrew: And guys, in the new movie—	
	Mrs. Kerry: Hold on. Jump in with a related story, Christian. (*3-second pause*) I …

TALK WITH ME

Student's Conversation	Adult Prompts
Christian: I've been to Disney World once. Taylor: Yeah, it's a great place, isn't it? Walsh: I rode on Space Mountain. Christian: Sometimes it's almost an hour in that line. Taylor: Yeah, I hate those lines, too. Walsh: Well, we were the first ones to get there, so my dad was like, "We're gonna go straight to Space Mountain." Christian: Do y'all like Thunder Mountain? Taylor: Yeah, that's my favorite ride. Walsh: We rode that in the dark the first time we went there. Taylor: Yeah, we did that, too. That's my favorite ride actually. Christian: Yeah, and we saw a statue of Walt Disney. Walsh: That's a famous statue. That's pretty cool. Andrew: So guys, what do you think the new *Star Wars* movie's gonna be about? Walsh: I don't know. Oh, speaking of movies coming out that we like, is anyone ready for the Ratchet and Clank movie? Will: Yeah and also the Sly Cooper movie. Walsh: Oh that's coming out next year. The Ratchet and Clank movie is coming out this year. Will: I know, because I can remember when it was announced or at least when I read about it. Henry: I think it might be like the super *Mario* movie. Walsh: No, it won't be. This is gonna be animated. Taylor: There's no way they could mess up as bad as the super *Mario* movie. Andrew: Yeah, my cousins got me that for Christmas, and I'm just like no. Just no. Walsh: It looks like they're gonna have it in the real setting. In the *Super Mario* movie, the stuff takes place in the city. Andrew: That was so stupid. Walsh: Peach wasn't even there. They didn't even look like plumbers. And what was up with the Goombas and Bowser? Andrew: I didn't even bother watching it because it was so bad, but my mom was like, "Oh, you should watch it. Your cousins think it's good." I'm like no they just know I'm a Super Mario fan. That's the only reason they got me it. Walsh: The little kids don't even pay attention to what makes a movie good.	
	Mrs. Kerry: All right. I'm gonna stop this one here. Let's look at how many questions, stories, and comments each of you had.

CHAPTER 2: RULES FOR IMPLEMENTING THE CONVERSATION FRAMEWORK

GAINING ADMINISTRATOR AND PARENT SUPPORT

Parents play an integral part when students are learning the steps in the Conversation Framework. With opportunities to converse with the student on a daily or regular basis, parents are able to track progress over time and ensure generalization of skills. If a student is going to participate in the Conversation Framework, is important for parents to be informed, which includes providing information about the steps, so they can understand the steps of the Conversation Framework, know which step is applicable in a given situation, and use strategies at home to support what is being taught through the Conversation Framework.

Appendix A includes a sample letter to parents. Please individualize this letter for your student's parent(s) or legal guardian based on the needs of the student.

As another important component to the effectiveness of the Conversation Framework, administrators in clinics as well as public or private schools rely heavily on professionals on their staff to understand and communicate the group size and group setting necessary for the work to be done. If a professional, such as a SLP or special education teacher, does not feel that he or she can accomplish the IEP or treatment goals effectively because of one of those factors, the concerns should be discussed with the administrator(s) as soon as possible so that creative alternatives can be explored.

1. Schedule a face-to-face meeting with your administrator.
2. Prepare key points for the conversation (see sample conversation below).
3. With administrator support, develop a collaborative plan of action.
4. If a parent or legal guardian is putting pressure on the adult to provide a service, yet permission has not been granted by the administrator, the professional should request that the parent or legal guardian set up a meeting with the administrator to discuss his or her concerns about the student's needs in more detail.

Sample Conversation for Professional to Gain Administrator Support

Thank you for providing support to allow me to work with my students. I believe we have a good team in place with good ideas.

I wanted to talk to you first because I am concerned about providing effective services for a few of our students. I currently am being asked to see ___ students within a ___ period of time ___ days per week because of their schedules. By doing this, I feel like I am not able to provide effective services for _____.

I was hoping we could collaborate to determine a plan of action that will work best for everyone.

Ideas for a Plan of Action

- Determine if someone else can provide services to ____ students during ____.
- Determine if a student's schedule can be changed.
- Check to see if the group duration can be shortened to create the opportunity for individual time before or after a group for students in need of individual services to focus on goals not addressed in a group setting (i.e., 20-minute group, 10-minute individual time).
- Check another student's schedule to see if he/she can participate to balance out the group.

CHAPTER 3
EMBEDDED SKILLS AND RELATED CONSIDERATIONS

In addition to the three fundamental steps of the Conversation Framework: identifying the topic, asking questions, telling stories, and making comments within 0-2 seconds, and bridging the topic, four skills are embedded in each step: active listening, tone, timing, and body language. While not the focus of this intervention, these skills are still very important. If a student struggles in one of these areas, he will still struggle in conversation even if he has mastered the other skills addressed in the Conversation Framework.

THE FOUR EMBEDDED SKILLS

Embedded skills here refer to skills taught throughout each conversation step within the Conversation Framework. The four embedded skills are (a) active listening, (b) tone, (c) timing, and (d) body language. None of these skills should be practiced in isolation. These play an essential role in successful conversations although not directly addressed.

Active Listening

Listening is more than hearing. Listening requires concentration on what is being said in an effort to understand and determine meaning. For the purposes of this book, *listening refers to the ability to attend and process what is being said*. Rather than being a prerequisite or an isolated step, listening is a requirement for all steps within the Conversation Framework. Many students with high-functioning autism spectrum disorder (HF-ASD) have difficulty with attending through active listening for a variety of reasons (please refer to Table 1.1). It is impossible to identify the topic without listening. Listening is a requirement for asking a relevant follow-up question or telling a story related to the topic, for these reasons listening is embedded into teaching the Conversation Framework.

Conversation Example With Prompts

The following example shows how prompts are used within an individual session. Throughout our sessions, we use a combination of verbal and visual prompts. The prompts are used to guide, redirect, refocus, and encourage students.

Age: 16 years old

Gender: Male

Group Size: 1 student (With Background Noise)

Conversational Goals:

Bailey – Embedded Skills (Listening With Background Noise)

Student's Responses	Adult Prompts
Bailey: It's hard to hear because he's like ... ah! (NOTE: He was talking about a group in the background doing a team-building game while his group was engaged in small talk. He said, "Ah," in frustration.)	
	Mrs. Kerry: You have to tune them out and focus. It's great practice.
Bailey: Alright, I'll try.	

Tone

Tone refers to the quality of the voice of the person speaking, including inflection and pitch. Volume and rate of speech are closely related to tone of voice. Because tone is often difficult to change, it is important to practice the appropriate tone during each stage of learning. How you say each word is just as important as what you say – sometimes more important, in fact; therefore, practice content and tone simultaneously. If a student with HF-ASD is working with a speech-language pathologist (SLP), for example, a discussion or written report between service providers may provide guidance in selecting specific prompts (verbal and visual) to incorporate consistently when embedding tone into the Conversation Framework.

Tips for Teaching Tone

- Prompt use of the correct tone
    - Model the inflection you want the individual to use
    - Model the pace of the words being spoken by speeding up or slowing down to change the emphasis of a specific word (which can also change the meaning of the word)
    - Discuss the emotion you are trying to convey
    - Use voice recordings for self-monitoring and feedback
    - Use voice recordings as a tool to show the difference between a word or phrase said two different ways

CHAPTER 3: EMBEDDED SKILLS AND RELATED CONSIDERATIONS

Timing

The switch that takes places between the speaker and listener in a conversation is called timing. Timing is critical. Indeed, one of the struggles that many individuals with ASD face in conversations is timing. Failure to understand and use proper timing in a conversation leads to awkward pauses, interruptions, talking at the same time as someone else, raising hand instead of jumping in, and changing of the topic of conversation at the wrong times. Timing within the Conversation Framework is learned through repeated practice and positive experience with each step. Visual supports for timing may be found in Appendices I and J.

> **Tips for Teaching Timing**
>
> Timing can be difficult to teach. Having awareness to know whether a situation is a conversation or whole-group listening can be tricky, especially if this does not come naturally to somebody. In whole-group listening, most students are taught to raise their hand before speaking. However, in conversation, raising your hand appears odd because the focus is on jumping in at the right time rather than somebody giving you permission to speak. Sometimes teaching the difference between the two can be as easy as telling students what situations might happen – conversation or whole-group listening and reminding them of the difference in behaviors expected. Appendix J provides a visual support that can be used in teaching awareness of timing in this area.

Body Language

Body language refers to nonverbal communication, including facial expressions, body posture, gestures, and eye movement. Appropriate body language makes a conversation believable. Body language can reflect an emotion – sympathy, sorrow, doubt, or enjoyment. It also conveys interest in people and in the conversation. Individuals with HF-ASD often have difficulty noticing, understanding, and using body language. Mirroring the student's body language can be an effective first step in teaching body language as it gives the student an opportunity to see what her body language looks like and, therefore, makes her more aware of how she comes across to others. When mirroring body language for a person with ASD, it is helpful to "freeze" the position or expression so the student has time to study it and "take it in." This turns the mirroring into a type of visual support – holding the information still in time.

THE "HIDDEN CURRICULUM"

Challenges with regard to the embedded skills outlined above are further compounded by the so-called "hidden curriculum – the ability to understand unstated rules within a social context (Myles, Trautman, & Schelvan, 2013). Many unstated rules vary with location, culture, relationship, gender, and emotional understanding. While most people generally pick up the nuances of the hidden curriculum very easily, these unwritten rules are challenging for individuals with HF-ASD and, therefore, need to be directly taught.

Location

Conversation involves many unstated rules depending on where you are when having the conversation. For example, when you are shopping in a grocery store, you typically have shorter conversations than if you are in a restaurant having dinner. The grocery store conversation is typically quick and to the point because people are busy shopping. However, when you are in a restaurant, the style of conversation is more intimate and specific because you have more time to talk. If you are at a sports event, such as a football game, the conversation will depend on how the game is going. If it is close, the crowd is probably loud and you won't be able to hear the person next to you. But if the game is dull and boring, you will have more opportunity to speak to the people around you.

Cultural Differences

Many unstated rules within conversations relate to race, religion, and culture, including speaking about differences as well as speaking to someone with differences. It is important to be aware of and honor cultural differences to avoid being perceived as offensive. It is not safe to assume that what is acceptable for one person is acceptable for another. For example, in some cultures, "yes" means "I hear you" rather than "I agree." Cultural differences may extend to dress, conversation style, and expected behavior.

Relationships

Relationships are fraught with unstated rules and social norms, influenced by roles, age, and closeness, all of which pose special challenges for individuals with HF-ASD.

Role

The role of each person within the relationship affects the relationship. For example, the role of teacher is different from the role of student. The role of the teacher is one of authority. In some cultures, the male in a relationship may be viewed as a provider or a leader and the female as a nurturer and caregiver. These roles may carry over into what is expected of each participant in a conversation.

Age

Age sometimes greatly affects the relationship but not always. For example, parents are almost always older than their children. A parent is often in authority. On the flip side, a boss may be younger than an employee. In this situation, age is not defining the role of the relationship, but it still affects the conversation.

Closeness

The depth or intimacy of a conversation depends on the comfort level or degree of closeness that exists between the partners in the relationship. When meeting someone for the first time, most people talk about general topics without going in depth. Conversations between those who have known each other for a long time such as a friend you have grown up with or a parent or sibling tend to be more deep or intimate.

Gender

While stereotyping others can be problematic, it is helpful for students with ASD to be taught general differences between the conversation of males and females. Typically, females talk more about people and emotions whereas males talk more about details and "random stuff." This general insight may help students with ASD to know what the expectations for conversation tend to be. However, it is important to know that these may be expectations, *NOT* rules. Each person should eventually be able to engage in conversations that are meaningful to him or her; however, it is helpful to know what the general expectations often are and to be able to "fit" those expectations.

CHAPTER 3: EMBEDDED SKILLS AND RELATED CONSIDERATIONS

Males in Conversation

Males can benefit from learning to talk about people and emotions, as it will assist with relationships with females. Males often talk about "stuff" and details. Males are more likely to have conversations about topics that might be described as "off color" or "crass." For example, two high school guys were talking about a video game. The dialogue included, *"I can get all 30 shots off ...They could blow off whatever piece ... If you are playing by yourself and you die, go up ... If you have multiple people, as long as one is still up there and alive ... one can get up there in time ... Go online, these videos online can show you how to do it ...Your only chances are coming up from underneath ...They turn around and you can blow off their head."*

Females in Conversation

Females tend to talk about people. For example, two young women who were in the same sorority were talking to each other at a restaurant. The dialogue included, *"Look at this picture ... This is when she fell on the ground on the dance floor ... I had to pick her up ... I was like, oh my God." ... "I like Abbie." ... "I sent Julie a picture of me and Casey and was telling her about last night."*

Body Position

Body position in conversation matters, especially in conversations between females. It is particularly important to pay attention to the difference between interested and uninterested body language. Most females in conversation will face each other, which signals that they are interested in what the other person has to say.

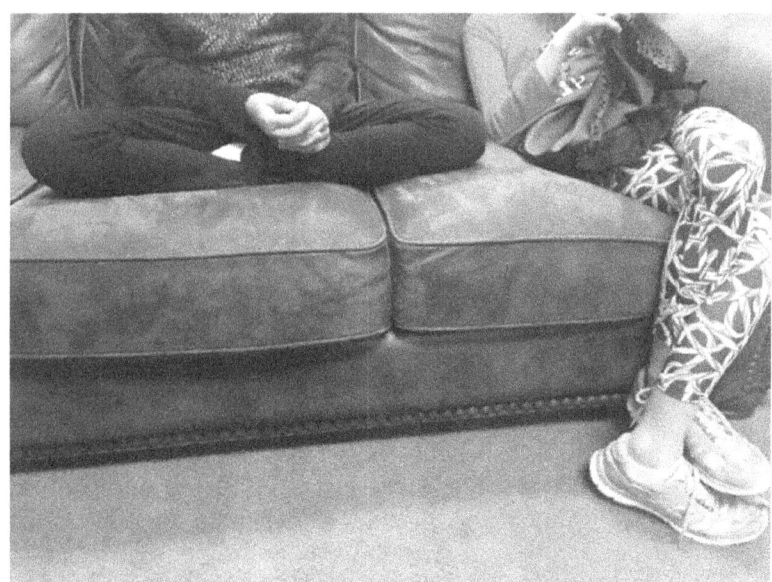

The girls are looking straight ahead. Their body position suggests that they are uninterested in each other.

31

TALK WITH ME

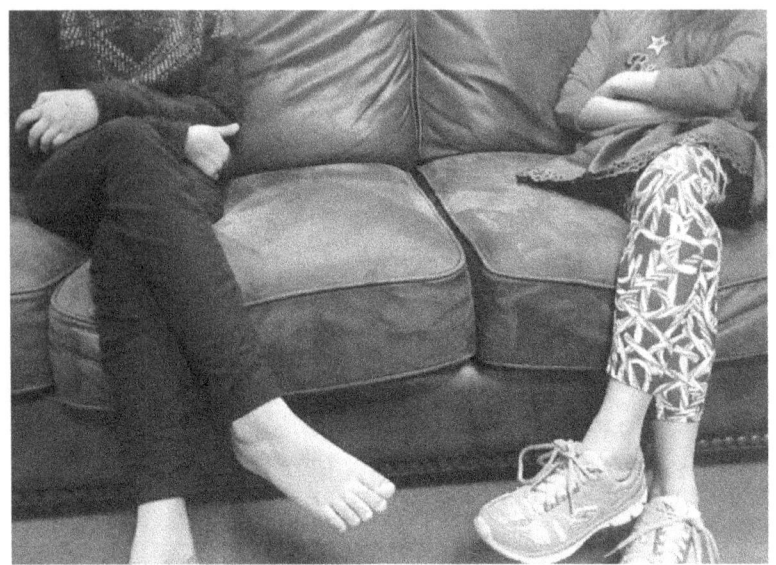

The girls have made adjustments to face each other; however, they have crossed arms, which generally signals being uncomfortable, cold, or "closed" – not open to mutual exchanges.

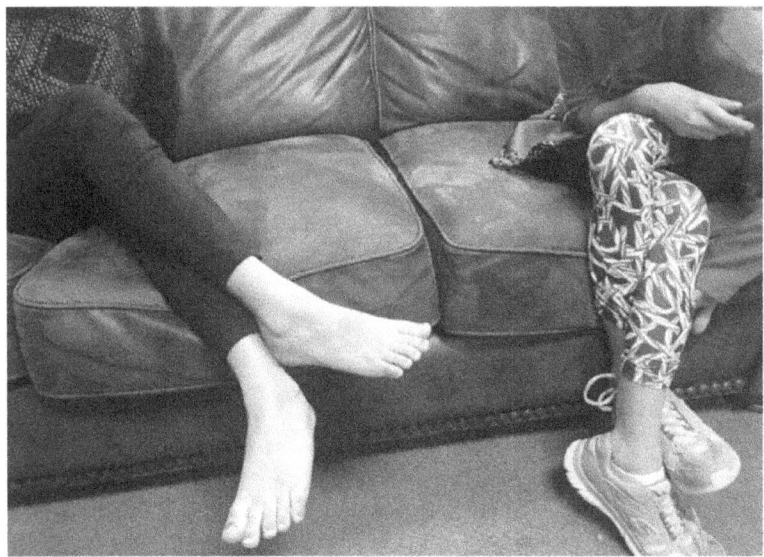

The girls are facing each other using their legs, shoulders, and bodies. They have uncrossed their arms to become more approachable and friendly.

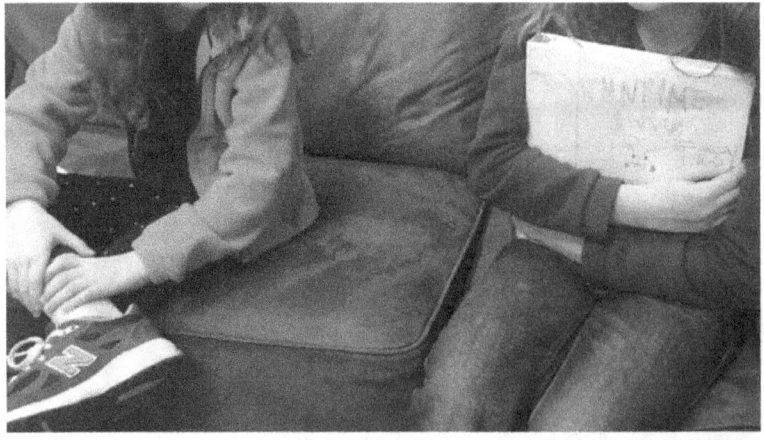

The girls are facing straight ahead and appear to be listening to someone across the room instead of each other. Although the girl on the left is making eye contact, this is body position is more consistent with interactions between males rather than females.

CHAPTER 3: EMBEDDED SKILLS AND RELATED CONSIDERATIONS

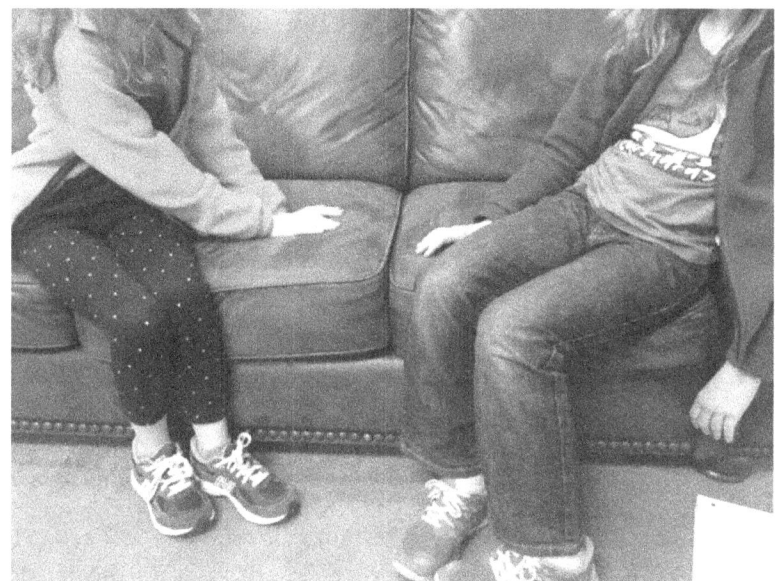

The girls are facing each other but are not using natural body language. The girl on the left is leaning in too much, which is making the girl on the right respond by leaning back so she has more personal space.

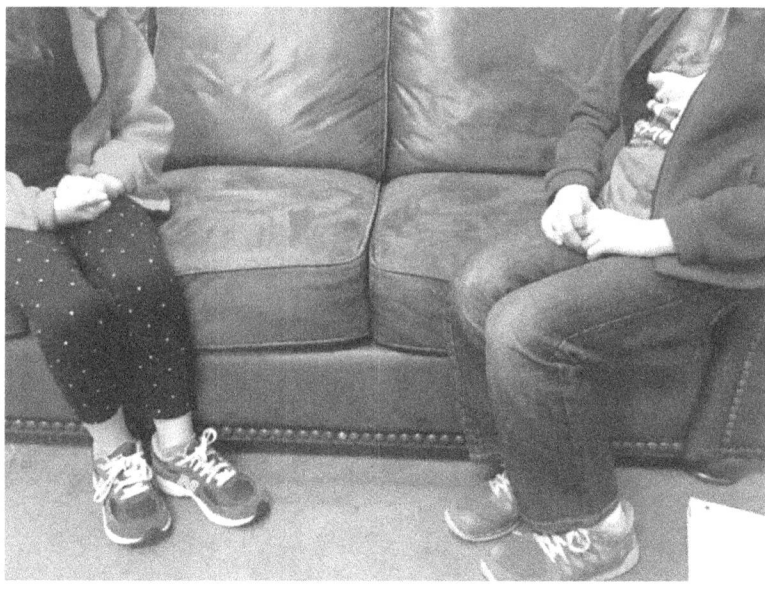

The girls are facing each other with their legs, shoulders, and bodies. Rather than having crossed arms, the girls have open body language. This is an ideal position for back-and-forth conversation.

Emotional Understanding

Being able to respond and relate to emotions in conversation is necessary in order to be able to interact effectively with others and build relationships. Emotional understanding helps be better employees, friends, and partners.

When the goal is to fit in, students must be able to match the intensity and type of emotion in a conversation to that of their peers. What makes this tricky is that statements often contain both facts and emotions. Sometimes the emotion is implied rather than directly stated. In an "emotional conversation," the conversation partner responds more to the emotions than the facts. Generally, neurotypical individuals are able to read the essence of a statement and immediately recognize when the emotion is more important to the conversation partner than the facts. This is more challenging for many individuals with ASD, who often need to be taught how to process this type of conversation.

The paragraph below contains excerpts from a conversation with strong emotional content. The conversation partner would be expected to recognize that the emotions being expressed are more important than the factual details.

> *Communication Partner 1: I've been so stressed out this past week because I got sick. I had to cancel so much stuff and move people around – super annoying. I hate being sick! I'm hoping to get over this pretty quickly. I was supposed to go and see my grandfather. Did I tell you that he got a new girlfriend ...*
>
> *Communication Partner 2: No. Didn't your grandmother just pass away ...*
>
> *Communication Partner 1: Well, it's been almost two years ...*
>
> *Communication Partner 2: Talk about some drama ... you will have to tell me about that. What do your parents think?*

If the communication partner responds to the comment "I've been so stressed out this past week because I got sick. I had to cancel so much stuff and move people around – super annoying" with, "Yes, I know. You canceled our meeting twice," he may appear to be insensitive or even selfish. A more fitting emotional alternative would be to say, "That's so awful. How are you feeling now?" Learning to recognize and respond to emotions increases opportunities for successful conversations.

Too often, active listening, tone, timing, and body language are taught as distinct skills, but practicing these skills in isolation is ineffective. When incorporated into teaching each step of the Conversation Framework, they become meaningful, helpful tools for "real-life" communication.

CHAPTER 4
THE THREE STEPS OF THE CONVERSATION FRAMEWORK

STEP 1: IDENTIFY THE TOPIC

"Identify the Topic" is the first step of the Conversation Framework because we must first listen to a conversation and identify the topic before we can ask relevant questions, tell related stories, or make appropriate comments – the other major components of participating in a conversation.

Identifying the topic focuses on what is being said. It includes the ability to recognize the overall theme or subject of the conversation as it emerges from the details of a conversation. As discussed in Chapter 1, this is often especially difficult for somebody with high-functioning autism spectrum disorder (HF-ASD), who may be able to attend to and process small details but has more difficulty than typically developing peers with seeing the big picture (Scherf et al., 2009) or identifying overall themes. Furthermore, people do not always say what they mean. What they mean to say is sometimes conveyed through innuendo (Haiman, 1998). In order to avoid alienation, individuals with HF-ASD must become skilled at finding the topic in real-life conversations with all of the subtleties that often entails.

> **Common Challenges**
>
> Common challenges that hinder the ability of individuals with HF-ASD to accurately identify the topic include:
>
> - **Forming categories.** They tend to interpret and form categories differently than others with specific attention to detail rather than big picture thinking (Church et al., 2010).
>
> - **Paying attention.** A high percentage exhibits symptoms of an attention deficit disorder (Volkmar et al., 2014).
>
> - **Lacking interest.** They are successful in attending to topics of high interest but pay little attention to topics of low interest to them (Gagnon & Myles, 2016; Tanidir & Mukaddes, 2014).

In education settings, identifying the topic is sometimes referred to as "stating the main idea." Identifying the main idea is required for academic subject areas, such as reading and language arts. Since most conversations are verbal (sign language may be used for conversation), identifying the topic is sometimes addressed under the category of listening comprehension in a school setting.

Two separate areas are required to correctly identify the topic: (a) identifying the overall topic, theme, or subject; and (b) identifying the weight of the conversation.

Identify the Overall Topic, Theme, or Subject of the Conversation

Categorical thinking allows individuals to process information by classifying similar information into groups or categories. Individuals with ASD were found to be less likely to use categorical thinking when making decisions in a task requiring them to find similarities between things (Church et al., 2010; Soulières, Mottron, Saumier, & Larochelle, 2007).

Conversation topics can be divided into the following categories: general topics, specific topics, or inferred topics. With younger students, inferred topics are typically not used in social settings.

General Topics

It is important to be able to identify the general category of the conversation because there is a main topic within every conversation – from the simplest to the most complex. The skill of identifying the topic must be directly taught to many individuals with HF-ASD.

In the list below, "Where You Are" refers to a person's location at any given moment. For example, the person may be at the library; thus, a general topic would be "starting a conversation about the library."

"Who You Are With" refers to those in a person's environment at any given moment. People in the setting often become the conversation topic. This is especially common when people are together and another person enters the room.

General Conversation Topics			
People/Lives	Weekend	Places	Family/Pets
School	TV Shows	Sports	Where You Are (right now)
Job	Movies	Food	Who You Are With (right now)
Hobbies/Interests	Music	Weather	Weird Things
Current Events	Electronics	Holidays	
News	Books	Vacations	

Specific Topics

As the complexity of a conversation increases, conversation topics become more specific. For example, within the general category of sports, the topic itself may be a specific player on a football team. In this example, sports is still the general topic; however, the specific topic is the player on a football team. The skill of identifying the specific topic must be directly taught to many high-functioning individuals with ASD.

Inferred Topics

Sometimes the true topic of a comment or conversation is hidden and must be inferred. Identifying these topics tends to be challenging for individuals with HF-ASD, who often interpret conversation in a literal manner. Clearly, this is problematic when the conversation partner assumes that the meaning, even though implied, is clear to the listener. Keep in mind that inferred topics can be an emotion, especially in conversations with a girl or woman. It is important to include conversations with inferred topics when working on this step of the Conversation Framework.

CHAPTER 4: THE THREE STEPS OF THE CONVERSATION FRAMEWORK

> **Conversation Example With Prompts**
>
> The following example shows how prompts are used within an individual session. Throughout our sessions, we use a combination of verbal and visual prompts. The prompts are used to guide, redirect, refocus, and encourage students.
>
> **Age:** 6 years old
>
> **Gender:** Male
>
> **Group Size:** 1 student (Individual Session)
>
> **Conversational Goals:** Matt – Step 1: Identifying the Topic
>
> **Strategy for Teaching the Conversation Framework**
>
> *Drill*
>
> *Fast-Paced Audio Recording*
>
> | Student's Conversation | Adult Prompts |
> |---|---|
> | | Mrs. Kerry: So tell me what a follow-up question is. |
> | Matt: A follow-up question is – I don't know. | |
> | | Mrs. Kerry: A follow-up question is a question about what someone just said. For example, if I said, "I'm going to eat a pickle today" and then said "Follow-up question," you'd ask me a follow-up question about what? |
> | Matt: Pickle. | |
> | | Mrs. Kerry: Yes, or me eating today or just today. Whatever I just said, you'd ask me about that. If I said that I saw the Alabama team logo on someone's hat just a little bit ago, you'd ask me what? |
> | Matt: Alabama logo. | |
> | | Mrs. Kerry: So, now what's the topic? |
> | Matt: Pickle. | |
> | | Mrs. Kerry: We've moved on from the pickle to ... |
> | Matt: Alabama logo. I hate football. | |
> | | Mrs. Kerry: You can hate football, but it's important that you are still able to talk about it and know that it's the topic. So, we're going to listen to a recording and you're going to do great identifying more topics. |

Identify the Weight of the Conversation

Another aspect of identifying the topic involves identifying the weight of what is being said as: light, medium, or heavy (see Appendix G). A light conversation is joking or silly in nature. A medium conversation is neutral, unemotional, or objective. A heavy conversation is serious. When working with younger children, rather than referencing light, medium, or heavy, it may be more practical to use two categories – joking/silly and serious.

The weight of the conversation is a key component to correctly identifying the topic and the two should be considered simultaneously and should be acquired from an early age.

The following examples of light and heavy topics illustrate what can happen when the difference between the two is not understood.

> *Claire said, "I'm not lying. At least one person finds a hair in their food every day. Most of the times, it's girls. I think with the girls it is probably their own hair if their hair is not in a ponytail. Never trust the food at my school."* (light)

> *Ava continued, "A boy named Brian had cancer; he came back to school today. He was wearing a hat because the cancer made him lose his hair. He now comes for half of the day to school, so he'll be coming half of the day as he rebuilds his strength." The group of five girls became silent and did not know what to say next.* (heavy)

What happened? Claire was telling a light story about her experiences. Ava identified the topic as hair without seeming to understand the weight of Claire's story and then told a story related to hair that she thought was similar to Claire's story; however, the weight of her story was heavy. With such a drastic change in the weight of the conversation, the conversation ended.

Considerations

The following should be considered with regard to the weight of the conversation: (a) developmental age, (b) group size and setting, (c) hesitation time, and (d) on- vs. off-topic comments and questions.

Developmental Age

Identifying the topic of conversation becomes a more complex process with age. For example, the skills required to be proficient in identifying the topic of conversation at 8 years old are different from the skills required to identify the topic of conversation at 18 years old. Therefore, even if the first step of the Conversation Framework is mastered at a young age, it still has to be addressed in the years to come. As a child ages, double meanings and sarcasm become increasingly common and topics become increasingly complex; as a result, previous steps of the Conversation Framework may need to be revisited as the student grows older.

Group Size and Setting

If a student has difficulty with identifying the topic of a conversation, this should be addressed in an individual or small-group setting. Fast-paced audio recordings (see pages 124-129) make it easier to replicate a conversation with peers in an individualized setting. If a student becomes embarrassed when guessing the topic in front of others, focus on this area in an individual rather than a group setting. This may include pulling the student to another space within the classroom away from the small group or to an alternate location. Conversation groups are generally more beneficial when all participants are working on identifying the topic or have worked on this skill previously and are somewhat familiar with the process.

Hesitation Time

Hesitation time, also known as response time or latency, refers to the time that it takes a person to retrieve the necessary information to be actively involved in a conversation. Because conversations occur rapidly, hesitation time matters. Some people need more time than others to get to the topic of a conversation, so hesitation time does not include the lead-up to the conversation because all conversations vary in complexity and length of time required to tell the story. For example, someone may give more background information to set up a story, thus, taking longer for the listener to identify the conversational topic.

A conversation about seeing a friend from school began with, *"My Dad usually goes grocery shopping on Saturday. Yesterday was Wednesday, but we ran out of milk – so my Dad took me with him to the store. We ended up getting some other things besides milk. While he was looking for milk I saw, Maria! Her hair is short now so I did not know who she was at first. I showed her my new phone."* The actual topic of the conversation – seeing a friend from school – came after a lengthy lead-up. The time to recognize the topic should not include the lead-up statements about shopping; it begins with the first sentence about Maria. Once asked to identify the topic, however, the student should be able to correctly identify and label the topic within less than 2 seconds.

On Topic vs. Off Topic

It can be difficult for someone with ASD to identify whether they are "on topic" or "off topic" because of challenges in the areas of perspective taking (such as difficulties with theory of mind, emotional understanding, and hidden curriculum) and language. If the person with HF-ASD changes the conversation to a topic of high interest, the new topic of high interest could potentially be perceived as "on topic" by the speaker with HF-ASD. It is not. Even though it is currently being discussed, it may be "off topic" from what the whole group was discussing.

Important rules to teach students about making on-topic comments:

- Try not to make an off-topic comment. If you must interrupt to say something off-topic, say, "Excuse me, sorry for interrupting …"
- To make an appropriate on-topic comment, wait for a pause in the conversation.
- Keep in mind:
  - One person talks at a time.
  - If you notice someone is talking at the same time as you, stop talking and let them finish.
  - If someone interrupts to add something on topic, it is okay.

STEP 2: BALANCE ASKING QUESTIONS, TELLING STORIES, AND MAKING COMMENTS WITHIN 0-2 SECONDS

The second step of the Conversation Framework is to "Balance Asking Questions, Telling Stories, and Making Comments Within 0-2 Seconds." For most typically developing individuals, balancing asking questions, telling stories, and making comments during conversation tends to emerge in a natural flow. For those with HF-ASD, this flow often remains imperceptible and confusing until they are directly taught to recognize the different parts of conversation and how to use them in the right combination; that is, achieve a balance between the various components.

> **Common Challenges**
>
> Common challenges that hinder the ability of individuals with HF-ASD to balance a conversation include:
>
> - **Processing speed**. They may process information at a slower pace than do typically developing peers (Goldstein et al., 2008).
> - **Atypical interpretation and formation of categories**. They may interpret and form categories differently than others, with specific attention to detail rather the big picture (Church et al., 2010).
> - **Challenges with sustaining attention**. A high percentage exhibits symptoms of an attention deficit disorder (Volkmar et al., 2014).
> - **Difficulty focusing on low-interest topics**. They may be successful in attending to topics of high interest but pay little attention to topics of low interest to them (Myles & Gagnon, 2016; Tanidir & Mukaddes, 2014).

Balancing a conversation requires knowing *what to say* in conversation. If somebody does not know what to say, he will most likely say the first thing that pops into his mind or say nothing at all.

Two different skills are required to balance a conversation using questions, stories, and comments within 0-2 seconds: (a) recognizing the parts of conversation: asking questions, telling stories, and making comments; and (b) balancing the parts of conversation. The Tally Mark Chart is used to support the development and use of this skill. Refer to pages 49-55 for instructions on how to use the Tally Mark Chart.

The Three Parts of Conversation

To become proficient in balancing a conversation requires first showing proficiency in each part of conversation: Asking Questions, Telling Stories, and Making Comments (see Appendices N and O). Typically, students with ASD are deficient in at least one of these areas. For example, Johnny may be good at asking questions but may need assistance in telling stories. Wu may be good at telling stories but may need assistance in asking questions about others.

The following describes Julia, who had difficulty with telling stories:

> *Julia started receiving services to improve her conversation skills when she was in the fourth grade. At that time, as measured by the Conversation Framework, she was only proficient in asking questions. In fact, she was almost too proficient at asking questions and often came across as interrogating others. Through informal assessments and observations in structured and unstructured settings, her IEP team agreed that she had a deficit in telling stories across all settings. Her stories were typically limited to one phrase or one sentence. While she was an intelligent and interesting student with good life experiences, she had difficulty communicating her thoughts to others in a story format.*

The following describes Santiago, who had difficulty with asking questions:

> *Santiago started social skills instruction at his school in the eighth grade. Across all settings, he told very long and energetic stories. The stories were often on topics that he was excited about, but that his listeners were less excited about. Santiago only asked questions if he was interested in what someone else was talking about; however, his interest in others' stories was rare. When he did ask questions, it was only for clarification on a detail that he was interested in rather than asking about the other person's experiences.*

CHAPTER 4: THE THREE STEPS OF THE CONVERSATION FRAMEWORK

Let's look at each part of a conversation in more detail, beginning with asking questions.

Asking Questions

It is difficult to have a conversation without asking questions. Questions allow us to get information, give information, and make others feel comfortable. Asking questions is difficult for some individuals with HF-ASD. In a research study examining the use of communication to get directions, individuals with ASD with low executive functioning abilities had difficulty asking effective questions to get the information needed. As a result, the ASD group required more turns in the conversation and asked less effective questions than the control group (Rajendran & Mitchell, 2006).

Common Challenges

Common challenges that hinder the ability of individuals with HF-ASD to ask questions include:

- **Understanding types of questions.** Failure to understand the types of questions and when they are used (Chin & Bernard-Opitz, 2000).
- **Identifying questions.** Difficulty formulating questions or asking shallow questions (Koegel, Koegel, Green-Hopkins, & Barens, 2010).
- **Lacking interest.** Not being interested in the topic discussed (White, Koenig, & Scahill, 2007).
- **Focusing on self.** Diverting the topic back to themselves or their experiences rather than focusing on others' experiences (White et al., 2007).
- **Requiring redirection.** Needing to be redirected to the task of asking questions (Laugeson, Frankel, Mogil, & Dillon, 2009).
- **Understanding others' perceptions.** Failure to understand how they are being perceived by others if they do not ask questions (Chin & Bernard-Opitz, 2000).

The following describes a student, Andrew, who had difficulty asking questions, even if all he had to do was to repeat a question that was provided for him:

> *The teacher said, "Say, Mrs. Kerry, do you like football?" Instead of asking that question, Andrew listed every reason that he did not need to ask that question, such as "I know you do not like football." During consultation with the parents about his difficulty asking questions, they connected his home behavior to this difficulty with asking questions. His father reported that Andrew threw away dishes that were difficult to clean and that he previously attributed Andrew's behavior to unwillingness to do this difficult task. Based on his new understanding of Andrew's overall difficulty with asking questions, his father's new hypothesis was Andrew's habit of throwing away dishes was due to Andrew's inability to ask a question to get help with washing dishes.*

Types of questions. There are three types of questions in conversations: (a) questions to start a conversation, (b) follow-up questions, and (c) reciprocal questions. All three are important for effective conversations.

Questions to start a conversation. A general question is often used to start a conversation, such as "What are you doing this weekend?" Individuals with HF-ASD should be able to generate questions on a variety of general topics as well as to recognize the difference between questions to use with someone you do not yet know and someone you know.

Table 4.1 lists sample topics for starting a conversation with people of varying ages.

Table 4.1
Sample Topics for Starting a Conversation

Question Topics for Starting a Conversation With School-Age People You Do Not Know	
Location	Ask about the activity or situation. • Is this the first time you have been to this camp? • What do you like to do at this park?
Who you are with	Ask about others who are there. • Do you know Samuel? • Are you in Jared's class, too?
Name	Ask for their name. • What's your name? • I'm ____(name). What's your name?
Grade/school	Ask for their grade and school. • What grade are you in? • What school do you go to?
Hobbies/interests	Ask about their interests. Try to find common interests. • What do you like to do on weekends? • What are you into? • Do you like ___ (something that you like)?
Where they live?	Ask a general question, not a street address. • What part of town do you live in? • Where do you live?

Question Topics for Starting a Conversation With Adults You Do Not Know	
Location	Ask about the activity or situation: • Do you come here a lot? • Have you been here before?
Who you are with	Ask about others who are there • Do you know Mrs. Holley? • How do you know Mrs. King?
Name	Ask for their name. • What's your name? • I'm ____(name). What's your name?
Job	Ask about their job. • Where do you work? • What do you do there?
Where they are from	Ask a general question, not a street address. • Where are you from? • Have you always lived here? • Where did you grow up?
Hobbies/interests	Ask about their interests. Try to find common interests. • What do you like to do on weekends? • Do you have a hobby?

CHAPTER 4: THE THREE STEPS OF THE CONVERSATION FRAMEWORK

Question Topics for Starting a Conversation With People You Know		
• People/lives • School • Job • Hobbies/interests • Current events • News • Weekend	• TV shows • Movies • Music • Books • Electronics • Sports • Weather	• Holidays • Vacations • Family/pets • Location • Who you're with • Weird things

Follow-up questions. A follow-up question is a question about what another person just said. Asking a follow-up question requires the ability to focus on the interests and thoughts of others and to connect to what another person is saying by asking a question to find out more information or show interest. This skill of perspective taking can be especially challenging for individuals with ASD.

Table 4.2 provides examples of follow-up questions for various topics.

Table 4.2
Sample Follow-Up Questions

	Examples of Follow-Up Questions
Conversation about rock climbing	• Statement of conversation partner: "I want to go rock climbing." • Follow-up question: "Have you ever been before?"
Conversation about homework	• Statement of conversation partner: "I have never had so much homework." • Follow-up question: "Is it all due this week?"
Conversation about tomorrow	• Statement of conversation partner: "Tomorrow is going to be great." • Follow-up question: "What's happening tomorrow?"
Conversation about books	• Statement of conversation partner: "I don't like reading fiction." • Follow-up question: "What kind of books do you like?"

Learning to ask follow-up questions helps the student talk with another person in a give-and-take manner. It is a necessary skill for having a true social interaction as opposed to using conversation as an avenue for repeatedly talking about one's own interests.

Conversation Example With Prompts

The following example shows how prompts are used within a natural conversation. Throughout our sessions, we use a combination of verbal and visual prompts. The prompts are used to guide, redirect, refocus, and encourage students.

Age: 8 - 9 years old (3rd- 4th grade)

Gender: Male

Group Size: 2 students

Conversational Goals

Peer 1 – Step 2: Asking Questions

Peer 2 – Step 2: Asking Questions

Strategy for Teaching the Conversation Framework

Natural Conversation

Students' Conversation	Adult Prompts
	Mrs. Kerry: I said, "I saw that someone had on a Kasey Kahne hat and he said he was just at a NASCAR race." Follow-up question.
Peer 1: I like Kasey Kahne.	
	Mrs. Kerry: So that would be a comment. What can you ask *me* about what I just said? A follow-up question.
Peer 1 & 2: *Pause*	
(Peer 1 raising his hand)	Mrs. Kerry: I said, "I saw that someone had on a Kasey Kahne hat and he said he was just at a NASCAR race." You'd say, "Hey, Mrs. Kerry." Okay put your hand down so I can hear you.
Peer 1: What's going on?	
	Mrs. Kerry: What's going on? What does that have to do with NASCAR? If you said, "Are you watching NASCAR *today*," that would have to do with NASCAR. But what's going on doesn't have anything to do with NASCAR unless you connect "what's going on" *with* "NASCAR."
Peer 1 & 2: *Pause*	
	Mrs. Kerry: Guys, I want you to ask *me* a question about NASCAR, so you'd say, "Mrs. Kerry, have you seen NASCAR?"
Peer 2: Mrs. Kerry, have you seen NASCAR?	
	Mrs. Kerry: I haven't, but my brother loves NASCAR.
Peer 2: I used to love cars a lot. I used to collect them.	
	Mrs. Kerry: What's your follow-up question for me?
Peer 2: Do you like NASCAR?	
	Mrs. Kerry: Good; that is a follow-up question about me. It's important to be able to ask questions about other people. I have a follow-up question for you on the topic of NASCAR. Have you seen a NASCAR race?

CHAPTER 4: THE THREE STEPS OF THE CONVERSATION FRAMEWORK

Closed- vs. Open-Ended Questions

A closed-ended question is a question that limits the type of response (i.e., "Do you like football?" elicits only a "yes" or "no" response). A closed-ended question is often helpful in determining interest in a general topic, but is limited in getting the respondent to engage and interact.

An open-ended question is a question that allows respondents to give as much or as little information as they would like in answering the question. Many times, open-ended questions encourage respondents to open up and talk about themselves or the topic.

Reciprocal questions. A reciprocal question is a specific type of follow-up question. It is basically the same question that a conversation partner just asked (or a close approximation). Reciprocal questions are an important part of many conversations. Table 4.3 lists examples of reciprocal questions.

Table 4.3
Sample Reciprocal Questions

	Examples of Reciprocal Questions
Two students find out they went to the same camp	• Original question: "What cabin were you in?" • Answer: "I was in Chickasaw cabin." • Reciprocal question: "Which cabin were you in?"
Two students are reading a novel about factions	• Original question: "What faction would you want to belong to?" • Answer: "Dauntless" • Reciprocal question: "What about you?"
Two students after watching a movie together	• Original question: "Who was your favorite character?" • Answer: I really liked Katniss." • Reciprocal question: "Yours?"
Two friends realize that they have both lived in Charleston.	• Original question: "When did your family live in Charleston?" • Answer: "When I was in elementary school." • Reciprocal question: "When were you there?"
Two people are getting to know each other.	• Original question: "Do you have pets?" • Answer: "I have two dogs." • Reciprocal question: "Do you have any?"
Two people are talking about each other's lives.	• Original question: "What are you doing this weekend?" • Answer: "Not much – I'm marching on Friday night. Other than that, nothing much because we were out of town last weekend." • Reciprocal question: "What about you?"

A teacher asked a student with ASD, "How are you?" The student's response was, "Good." He did not ask about the teacher, who then asked, "Do you care how I'm doing?" The student's response was "No." Because the teacher recognized the underlying challenges of this student with ASD, she did not take offense but continued by saying, "You do not have to care about how someone is feeling, but you do need to ask someone how they are doing anyway." The teacher went over it again by saying "When someone says 'How are you?," you should always follow up with 'Good, how are you?' It only takes a second, and it is what is expected."

This example demonstrates the importance of reciprocal questions. Most people know when a reciprocal question is the next step in a conversation. However, mindblindness, the difficulty recognizing thoughts and feelings of others, may affect the ability to ask a reciprocal question (Chin &

Bernard-Opitz, 2000; De Rosnay, Fink, Begeer, Slaughter, & Peterson, 2014). If the reciprocal question is not asked, an awkward pause may occur. Most individuals with ASD care about the person they are talking to but may not understand the role of reciprocal questions in showing their respect for and interest in others and, therefore, need to be directly taught.

Telling Stories

Life is a series of stories. We become engaged when someone mentions the word *story* in anticipation of learning something interesting or being entertained. Stories are the backbone of our history books, childhood memories, and family heritage. Stories allow us to convey an emotion, give information, and entertain others.

Through telling stories about plans, experiences, thoughts, and emotions, we build emotional connections with others. Because people with HF-ASD often do not notice these emotions, they have a harder time developing emotional connections through conversation. In a research study designed for high-functioning children with ASD, researchers found that the ability to tell stories was linked with emotional understanding in developing shared experiences and deeper relationships (Losh & Capps, 2003).

Common Challenges

Common challenges that hinder individuals with HF-ASD in telling engaging stories include:

- **Story concepts.** Failure to understand the concept of stories and what a story consists of (Diehl, Bennetto, & Young, 2006).
- **Connecting emotions to stories.** Difficulty with connecting an emotion to stories, so stories sound bland, boring, and emotionless (Losh & Capps, 2003).
- **Organizing.** Difficulty organizing a story in a logical order because of challenges in executive functioning, sometimes resulting in stories that are confusing to others (Diehl et al., 2006).
- **Considering the needs of the listener.** Failure to consider what background information the listener needs in order to understand the story being told or to consider whether the listener is interested in the story. This is related to failure to recognize or understand the perspective of others (Rehfeldt, Dillen, Zioemek, & Kowalchuk, 2010).
- **Explaining answers.** Difficulty explaining an answer correctly (Loukusa et al., 2007).

Types of stories. There are three general types of stories: sequential, informational, and emotional. Stories can be a mixture of several of these. All are important for effective conversation. In addition to the types of stories, the stories can be categorized as follows: (a) stories to start a conversation and (b) related stories.

Sequential stories. Sequential stories are told using details in the same order as something that happened, similar to a timeline. They can include details from a 5-minute event or from events spanning 100 years.

> *I went hunting with my dad and Mr. Joe. We saw a few bucks, but Mr. Joe said not to shoot them because they would mature and get bigger for next year. Thomas and I just watched turkeys in a field and rode four-wheelers. We had dinner on the campfire. Dad cooked it.*

CHAPTER 4: THE THREE STEPS OF THE CONVERSATION FRAMEWORK

Informational stories. Informational stories are told in a way that describes something; they can be sequential or nonsequential. If nonsequential, the stories may use information from past and present events without attention to sequential order.

> *The Kingda Ka is the world's tallest roller coaster. It goes 456 feet in the air and 128 mph. It's located at Six Flags in New Jersey.*

Emotional stories. Emotional stories are stories that convey an emotion, whether or not the emotion is directly stated or implied. In order for the listener to feel an empathetic response to an emotional story, the person talking must be able to deliver the story using the embedded skills body language, tone, and facial expressions (see page 29) that are appropriate to the emotion of the story.

> *I just found out that I am moving to New York and starting a new job! I'm so excited and cannot wait to move. I went up there to visit last month and found an apartment, so everything is set. My parents are going to ride up there with me to move all of my stuff.*

Reasons to tell a story. Stories may also be categorized based on the reason for telling them into (a) stories to start a conversation and (b) related stories.

Stories to start a conversation. Stories to start a conversation are just that – stories that are used to start a conversation with someone. Most stories in this category are about either something unusual that happened, current news, or a current situation in someone's life. This type of story typically includes phrases such as "You won't believe what happened to me today ..." or "Did you hear about ...?" For example, someone might say, "You won't believe what I saw on my way to work ... there was an 18 wheeler towing a tank ... it was pretty awesome."

Related stories. Related stories include stories that are related to what is being said. Related stories can be any type of story (sequential, informational, or emotional) but should always have the same weight and topic (see pages 37-39) as the conversation. Related stories can include opinions on a main topic (see Appendix K), such as providing an opinion about what you think about a political candidate, something happening in the news, or something that a coworker did. Opinions – for or against something or someone – can be embedded into a story. Opinions can also express like or dislike for something or someone.

> ***First Person's Story to Start a Conversation:*** *You will never believe what happened to me the other day. I was in the grocery store and saw some dude just lying on the ground by the entrance. He was lying there the entire time I was in there.*
>
> ***Second Person's Comment****: That's so weird.*
>
> ***Second Person's Question:*** *Was he ok?*
>
> ***First Person's Response:*** *Yeah. I asked if he was ok and he said that he was just a little winded, so he was taking a rest.*
>
> ***Second Person's Related Story:*** *Speaking of weird things, at school the other day, a stray dog walked into the building and into a classroom before anyone noticed it. Someone had left the door open, and it let itself in.*

> **Conversational Experiences**
>
> To join a conversation, students need things to talk about. In order to obtain stories to tell, students need to do things such as:
>
> - Look up school events
> - Participate in after-school activities
> - Participate in clubs
> - Stay current with state sports teams
> - Watch popular TV shows
> - Watch movie trailers for upcoming movies
> - Watch the news
> - Search online for current news
> - Listen to music
> - Read books, magazines, and news articles

> **Story Toppers**
>
> A "one-upper" or "story topper" is slang for someone who tops every story with an even better version of the story just told. A "one-upper" or "story topper" is often perceived as a sign of wanting to be the center of attention. People who are story toppers do not let others have the spotlight, come across as self-centered, and appear to have little interest in the stories of others. Warn students about one-upping their conversation partners.

Making Comments

Comments – short phrases used to keep a conversation going – are the most frequently used part of conversation. Making a comment is the quickest way to participate in a conversation and the easiest way to show people that you are interested in what they have to say. Comments encourage others to keep their story going and let others know that you are listening to what they are saying.

> **Common Challenges**
>
> Common challenges that hinder the ability of individuals with HF-ASD to make relevant comments include:
>
> - **Understanding comments.** Failure to understand the concept of comments and their purpose (Franke & Durbin, 2011).
> - **Taking perspectives.** Failure to know the perspective of others and why a comment would be needed to show interest or participate in the conversation (Peterson, Garnett, Kelly, & Attwood, 2009).
> - **Timing.** Not knowing how to time a comment correctly (Stribling, Rae, & Dickerson, 2009).
> - **Showing interest**. Not having interest in the conversation (Wang & Spillane, 2009).

The following describes a student, Raj, who almost exclusively used one-word comments in conversation:

> *Wayne asked Raj, "So what are you doing this weekend." Raj said, "Nothing." To keep the conversation going, Wayne said, "Are you going to play video games?" Raj answered, "Yea." Wayne then asked, "What video games do you like?" Raj said, "RPG." At this point, the pressure to keep the conversation going was on Wayne, and he was beginning to lose interest. He could not get a back-and-forth conversation going with Raj. He was trying to ask open-ended questions to get Raj talking; however, Raj was only using one-word or phrase response comments.*

CHAPTER 4: THE THREE STEPS OF THE CONVERSATION FRAMEWORK

Types of comments. There are four types of comments: (a) reflex comments, (b) empathetic comments, (c) response comments, and (d) satirical comments.

Reflex comments. Reflex comments are stated as a spontaneous reaction to something that happened or something that was said. For example, Max told Syd that Lucy is pregnant. Amy overheard the statement. She said, "At her age?" This type of comment typically communicates an honest opinion without filtering the social context of whether or not the comment would be socially appropriate.

Empathetic comments. Empathetic comments express care, interest, or compassion with regard to something that is happening or being said. Tireeq said, "I don't want to go to work today." Rather than asking why, Ashley said, "Sorry." This type of comment typically communicates interest and care; however, the comments do not necessarily reflect the intentions of the person making the comment.

When learning to make empathetic comments, we need to relate emotion in a comment. The following is an example of a sentence and a range of responses that focus on the emotional content.

I didn't make the tennis team this year.
- That's awful.
- Sorry to hear that.
- Can't believe that happened.
- How frustrating.

Response comments. Response comments are stated as an on-topic response to a question. As such, they are important parts of a conversation. Sarah asked, "Julie, what have you been doing today." Rather than telling a story, Julie said, "Not much."

Satirical comments. Satirical comments include the use of irony, sarcasm, or ridicule. Many people with ASD tend to think in a concrete or literal manner; therefore, they may have difficulty interpreting or using satirical comments.

Satirical comments are often used to make light of a bad situation. To one of his buddies, Miller said, "I'm definitely living the happily ever after." The reality was that he was not "living happily ever after" but was on the verge of breaking up with his girlfriend. Sarcastic comments made between two friends may appear to be negative but can be used in a joking tone where both friends interpret the humor of the comment. Although there are many positive uses for satirical comments, this type of comments can come across as mean or unkind if done incorrectly or if the comment is ill intended.

Balancing the Conversation Using the Tally Mark Chart

The Tally Mark Chart is a visual representation of the parts of conversation, asking questions, telling stories, and making comments, with each tally mark representing one question, one story, or one comment. The overall goal of the Tally Mark Chart is to help conversation partners balance the questions, stories, and comments first within the individual's contributions to the conversation (equal representation of questions, stories, and comments) and then with everyone else within the conversation group (equal representation of questions, stories, and comments as everyone else).

Balancing Conversation With Two People

In a conversation between two people, it is important for both people to talk. Both people should be asking questions to learn more about what the other person is saying. Both people should be sharing stories with the other person. Both people should be making comments to show interest.

Below is an example, first of an unbalanced conversation between two people and then of a balanced conversation.

Unbalanced

	Asking Questions	Telling Stories	Making Comments
Person 1	-	⊥⊥⊥⊥	IIII
Person 2	IIII	I	IIII

Balanced

	Asking Questions	Telling Stories	Making Comments
Person 1	IIII	IIII	⊥⊥⊥
Person 2	III	IIII	III

Balancing Conversation With a Small Group

In a balanced conversation between a small group of people, typically three to five, each person should contribute questions, stories, and comments on topic for the conversation to be balanced.

Below is an example, first of an unbalanced conversation within a small group of people and then of a balanced conversation.

Unbalanced

	Asking Questions	Telling Stories	Making Comments
Person 1	-	-	III
Person 2	-	⊥⊥⊥ II	-
Person 3	-	-	I
Person 4	IIII	I	-

Balanced

	Asking Questions	Telling Stories	Making Comments
Person 1	II	II	III
Person 2	IIII	I	III
Person 3	III	III	III
Person 4	III	II	III

CHAPTER 4: THE THREE STEPS OF THE CONVERSATION FRAMEWORK

Balancing Conversation With a Large Group

In a large group of people, typically six or more, the ability to participate by telling stories may be limited because it is difficult for everyone to be able to tell a story on each topic. In a large group, it is also difficult for people to balance the questions, stories, and comments with themselves because of the large number of people who need to speak. Instead, questions, stories, and comments should be balanced with each person in the conversation. That is, generally, everyone in the conversation should tell about the same number of stories and ask about the same number of questions.

Below is an example, first of an unbalanced conversation between members within a large group and then a balanced conversation.

Unbalanced

	Asking Questions	Telling Stories	Making Comments
Person 1	-	III	-
Person 2	-	-	I
Person 3	III	IIII	HTT I
Person 4	II	-	HTT HTT
Person 5	IIII	-	-
Person 6	-	-	HTT II
Person 7	I	II	III
Person 8	HTT IIII	HTT III	HTT HTT

Balanced

	Asking Questions	Telling Stories	Making Comments
Person 1	IIII	I	HTT I
Person 2	II	I	IIIII
Person 3	I	II	IIII
Person 4	II	I	HTT
Person 5	III	I	IIII
Person 6	II	II	HTT
Person 7	II	0	IIII
Person 8	II	I	IIII

Conversation skills are often taught in artificial exercises and, therefore, do not become natural and smooth-flowing. Because many individuals with HF-ASD have difficulty with using context to understand social interactions (Patel, Preedy, & Martin, 2014), it is imperative for them to practice conversation in the context of real conversation settings. The Conversation Framework does just that by moving away from strategies used in other social skills programs, such as contrived communication cards that are out of context.

Conversation Example With Prompts

The following example shows how prompts are used within a natural conversation. Throughout our sessions, we use a combination of verbal and visual prompts. The prompts are used to guide, redirect, refocus, and encourage students.

Age: 12 - 18 years old

Gender: Female

Group Size: 7 students

Conversational Goals

    Chloe – Step 2: Balancing the Conversation (On Topics of Non-Interest)
    Kristen – Step 2: Balancing the Conversation (Without Dominating)
    Corey – Step 2: Balancing the Conversation (Including Asking Questions About Others)
    Hannah – Step 2: Balancing the Conversation (Including Asking Questions About Others)
    Samya – Step 2: Balancing the Conversation (Including Initiation on Jumping Into the Conversation With a Question, Story, or Comment)
    Julia – Step 2: Balancing the Conversation (Including Telling a Story with Emotional Connection)
    Megan – Step 2: Balancing the Conversation (Including Asking Follow-Up Questions)

Strategy for Teaching the Conversation Framework

Natural Conversation

Students' Conversation	Adult Prompts
Chloe: We used to have a goldfish, but she died.	
Kristen: The goldfish died?	
Hannah: We had a beta fish, then my brother got like three other fish. Beta fish like to be alone. He got three other fish. All of the other fish died before the beta fish. We had a bunch of fish before that. Now we are not getting any more fish, but we have a dog.	
Megan: What kind of dog?	
Hannah: My dog is a mix between a greyhound and a German Shepherd.	
Kristen: Is it a boy or girl?	
Hannah: Girl.	
Megan: What's her name?	
Hannah: Josie.	
Corey: You've had her for a while, right?	
Hannah: Yes. How long have you had your cats?	
Corey: A long time. I don't remember getting them. My mom said they are 15.	
	Mrs. Kerry: Samya, do you know when to time it right to jump in? Watch my finger, and I'll help you. You'll have to wait for a quick pause, but be ready to tell a related story.

CHAPTER 4: THE THREE STEPS OF THE CONVERSATION FRAMEWORK

Corey: I like my cats.	
	Mrs. Kerry: (*gesture prompt for Samya to jump into the conversation*)
Samya: I don't have any pets. I do want a pet. Kristen: What kind of pet do you want? Samya: A dog. Chloe: What kind of dog? Samya: A poodle. Kristen: Megan, do you have any pets? Megan: I have one cat named Elijah. Chloe: My family is getting a new dog. You probably remember that my old dog, Rose, died, so we are ready to get a new dog.	
	Mrs. Kerry: Bridge this conversation into something else. Speaking of …
Megan: Speaking of pets …	
	Mrs. Kerry: It could be speaking of animals, or speaking of things that I enjoy.
Megan: Speaking of animals, I wanted a real chicken for Christmas. Corey: You got one? Megan: I didn't get a real one. I got a stuffed animal. It was the next best thing. Corey: I was going to say that, well, for Christmas, I got stuffed animals. I got one from my brother and one from Santa. Also, I got Christmas money. My mom took me to a store, and I got one of those really big ones. Hannah: I love those. Corey: Yea, my brother got one, and I wanted one. Julia: Speaking about stuffed animals. I have two things to say about stuffed animals. First, I gave away all of my stuffed animals and toys because I've outgrown them. And second, I was watching this movie – well, TV show – called *Futurama*. This college girl intern girl named Amy was trying to get this key out of a stuffed animal thing, and she kept getting stuffed animal. Girls: Laughed.	
	Mrs. Kerry: Speaking of weird things, today I walked into the other room. There was a cooler in there from before the holidays. I was thinking Capri Suns. It was a lot of moldy fruit and it smelled treacherous. I went to put it in the dumpster. It started dripping by my feet. When I did it, it banged from the dumpster.

53

Megan: What? Chloe: What happened? Kristen: She said that a nasty cooler dumped on her. Hannah: So there's this girl in my drama class, and she somehow was opening a bag, and she cut her hand with a potato chip. I don't know how she did that. Corey: Did she have to go to the hospital? Hannah: She had to get stitches. Julia: Speaking of weird things, I have the weirdest thing happen to me. My acting teacher from Children's Dance Foundation, her son, he was running really fast, and (in the toddler room), he fell on a train and flipped over and got hurt. It was something that happened when he was 2 or 3.	
	Mrs. Kerry: Be sure to think of something current if you can.
Kristen: I've told y'all about this. I told y'all when we were at show choir, and I tripped. I tripped over a cord. Julia: Oh wow. Corey: You slipped on the fan? Chloe: Did you fall on the floor? Julia: Were you okay? Kristen: Yes.	
	Mrs. Kerry: Don't look at me. Look at them.

If tracking the conversation using the Tally Mark Chart for each question (Q), story (S), and comment (C), the chart would look like this:

	Q	S	C
Chloe	III	I	I
Kristen	IIII	I	II
Corey	IIII	II	II
Hannah	I	II	IIII I
Samya			III
Julia	I	II	I
Megan	III	I	II

The following considerations are important when setting up groups. In addition, Appendix X includes a description of various types of group participants, from those you rarely say anything to those who monopolize the conversation and how to deal with them.

Considerations

Age of Development

It is never too early to start practicing asking questions, telling stories, and making comments. Although you would not practice balancing conversation until elementary school, students can begin learning the parts of conversation (how to ask a question, how to tell a story, how to make a comment) in preschool.

CHAPTER 4: THE THREE STEPS OF THE CONVERSATION FRAMEWORK

Group Size and Setting

If a student has difficulty in one of the three parts of conversation, the skill should be addressed in an individual or small-group setting. Group size and background noise matter. It is important that the group size reflects the needs of each individual. Start with the setting that would be the easiest for the student. When he masters that part of conversation in the easiest setting begin to introduce new more challenging settings in which to practice the skill.

It is typically easier to work on making comments in a group setting, because they are largely contingent on timing. Practicing conversation in various situations will help the student to generalize skills more easily.

The following is a list of typical group sizes and settings for conversation.
- 1 peer or adult
- 2 peers
- 3 - 5 peers
- 6 - 8 peers
- 8+ peers
- Without background noise
- With background noise (constant)
- With background noise (changing)
- Unstructured setting (hallway transition, recess, lunch)
- Structured setting (classroom)
- Sitting
- Standing

Once an individual joins a large group, he should already be familiar with the terms and concepts of the Conversation Framework and be able to give an accurate response to a prompt within 0-2 seconds hesitation time. Initially, success in large groups might require use of a predetermined nonverbal gesture or cue to remind the student to ask a follow-up question or make a comment. This cue will allow the student to be successful in remembering what he is supposed to do without becoming the negative focus of the large group's attention if his name is repeatedly called aloud. If conversation services are taught in a larger group setting, the student may not receive the amount of repeated practice or positive experience necessary to master the parts of conversation.

If you have limited access to peer groups, consider utilizing fast-paced voice recordings or video from a fast-paced conversation to mimic the type of conversation the student would hear in peer groups. Recordings can be effective at teaching the basic skills but cannot replace a peer group. See pages 124-129 for information on using fast-paced audio recordings.

Hesitation Time

The skill for generating questions, stories, and comments must be developed to the point that it can be performed very rapidly – within 2 seconds. The latency of the responses is important. If it takes somebody 10 seconds to make an appropriate comment, she will most likely become excluded from the conversation because the conversation partner will assume that she is not interested in or does not understand what was said. Instead, the conversation partner is likely to respond to another member of the group who contributed to the conversation in a timely manner – within 2 seconds.

Because many teachers teach conversation in a structured or isolated setting, the balance of conversation is typically not addressed. For example, a student who asks too many questions may have been "over-taught" to ask questions, whereas a student who tells too many stories may have been "over-taught" to tell stories.

STEP 3: BRIDGE THE TOPIC

When first developing the concept of the Conversation Framework, I thought that it ended with questions, stories, and comments. In fact, I always told clients those components were "all you do" in conversation. However, when I noticed that my clients were mastering the skills that I taught them (questions, stories, comments), yet not maintaining a longer conversation, I wondered, "What am I missing?" The answer is: the concept of bridging the topic, thus extending the length and variety of the conversation. Many clients thought they had to stay "on topic" even if the topic had completely ended.

> *"You're off topic," Miles said to his peer. As the group leader, I responded, "Sometimes people change the topic and it flows into a new topic." This was something this group had not worked on before, so I was trying to explain how changing the topic was okay in this instance. Miles continued, "We were not talking about a car show; we were talking about Barber Speedway. George started talking about a car show and I'm not interested in car shows." I said, "What could you say to him if you wanted to change the topic from car shows?" Miles responded, "I don't know." At that point, Miles needed tools to maneuver between topics.*

Once the other areas of the Conversation Framework have been mastered, the final step is to learn how to bridge topics from one topic to another without a drastic change.

Despite his own enjoyment of talking about topics of high interest, when somebody talks about one preferred interest in a lot of detail it can be boring for others in the conversation. Bridging the topic allows us to guide the conversation from one topic to a new and interesting topic. It is a skill that creates flow to a conversation through the use of changing categories and is vital in maintaining a longer conversation. Advantages of knowing how to successfully bridge the topic also include having the power to change the direction of the conversation and not feeling stuck on one topic, especially when the topic is non-preferred.

While bridging the topic allows us to navigate between topics, alone this skills does not enable us to maintain or go in depth on a topic. If we only bridged topics during a conversation, it would probably sound like "Speaking of beaches, I went to the beach. Speaking of beaches, my mom is from the beach. Speaking of your mom, I have not talked to my mom. Speaking of talking to people, I do not like the telephone." Thus, using Step 3 of the Conversation Framework exclusively does not lead to fluency in conversation. It is the balance of using Steps 1, 2, and 3 that creates conversational balance and fluency.

Bridging the Topic

A social group practiced bridging the topic using something they had talked about in small groups. Not surprisingly, they chose to bridge off of the topic of video games.
- Speaking of hobbies, I like to play with Legos. (*Prompted to change to a question.*)
- Speaking of hobbies, does anyone like Legos?
- Speaking of hobbies, what do you guys like to do?
- Speaking of the weekend, what do you during your weekend?
- Speaking of electronics, I heard the new iPhone 8 was coming out.
- Speaking of the weekend, do any of you like to fish?
- Speaking of video games, what other video games do you like to play? (*Prompted to change to a different topic.*)
- Speaking of video games, what other electronics do you like to play?
- Speaking of video games, I heard they are making a new Nintendo Switch. (*Prompted to change to a different topic.*)
- Speaking of weekends, what are you doing this weekend?
- Speaking of your brother (*said he played video games with him often*), is he older or younger than you?
- Speaking of video games, who's excited about the new video games? (*Prompted to change to a different topic.*)

CHAPTER 4: THE THREE STEPS OF THE CONVERSATION FRAMEWORK

Conversation Example With Prompts

The following example shows how prompts are used within an individual session. Throughout our sessions, we use a combination of verbal and visual prompts. The prompts are used to guide, redirect, refocus, and encourage students.

Age: 10 - 12 years old

Group Size: 2 students

Conversational Goals

Peer 1 – Step 3: Bridging Topics

Peer 2 – Step 3: Bridging Topics

Strategy for Teaching the Conversation Framework

Conversation Topics List

Students' Conversation	Adult Prompts
Peer 1: Did anyone go outside today?	
Peer 2: I went into my grandparents' backyard, took my bb gun and took out the golf cart. I only rode as far as my grandparents would let me.	
	Mrs. Kerry: What's the topic?
Peer 2: Forest.	
	Mrs. Kerry: Look on your list.
Peer 2: Weekend.	
	Mrs. Kerry: What else?
Peer 2: Let me remember. How am I supposed to remember this? Vacation?	
	Mrs. Kerry: Not a vacation unless you took a vacation from school. What else could it be?
Peer 1: Weekend.	
	Mrs. Kerry: Yes, you guys have said that.
Peer 1: Lives.	
	Mrs. Kerry: Yes. What else?
Peer 1: I don't know.	
	Mrs. Kerry: You've got this.
Peer 1: Holiday. Family.	
	Mrs. Kerry: Speaking of …
Peer 1: Speaking of family, do you have brothers and sisters?	
	Mrs. Kerry: Yes. That's a great bridge. You got from weekend to family.

> **Common Challenges**
>
> Common challenges that hinder individuals with HF-ASD in bridging topics include:
>
> - **Using one topic.** They tend to talk on one topic for too long (Wing, 1981).
> - **Forming categories.** They interpret and form categories differently than others with specific attention to detail rather than the big picture (Church et al., 2010).
> - **Lacking flexibility.** Many are rule-bound or have difficulty changing topics due to deficits in flexibility and organization (Kenworthy et al., 2005; Kleinhans, Akshoomoff, & Delis, 2005).

As discussed earlier, conversations can be categorized into general topic areas such as weekend, sports, current events, and family (see page 36). Many people base decisions and changes in conversation on how they perceive the conversation topic. At times, we all choose to take a conversation in another direction, thus changing the topic. It is the understanding of topics that leads to creating an effective flow to the conversation without an abrupt topic change. Bridging the topic to new and related conversation topics requires flexibility, problem solving, and planning. There are two ways to bridge the topic: (a) expanding the topic and (b) condensing the topic.

Expanding the Topic

Expanding the topic focuses on moving the conversation from where you are to where you want it to go by identifying new conversation topics. The newly identified topics must be different yet related to the original topic. To demonstrate mastery of bridging topics, an individual must show proficiency in identifying the topic and effectively bridging the topic to another related topic using a question, story, or comment. Scripts such as "Speaking of …" and "That reminds me of …" may be used to help an individual gain proficiency in this area.

Condensing the Topic

Condensing the topic focuses on gradually moving the conversation from one given topic to another though the discovery and identification of a common category. The common category is typically a broader, more general, category. For example, hobbies and sports both fit into "things you do." In that instance, you'd be condensing the categories of hobbies and sports into "things you do." Many times the common category is inferred rather than directly stated. Being aware of the common category is a key skill in creating a flow within a conversation.

> **Conversation Example With Prompts**
>
> The following example shows how prompts are used within a natural conversation. Throughout our sessions, we use a combination of verbal and visual prompts. The prompts are used to guide, redirect, refocus, and encourage students.
>
> **Age:** 13 - 15 years old
>
> **Group Size:** 3 students
>
> **Conversational Goals:**
>
> >   Walsh – Step 3: Bridging Topics
> >
> >   Pearce – Step 3: Bridging Topics
> >
> >   Henry – Step 3: Bridging Topics
>
> **Strategy for Teaching the Conversation Framework:**
>
> >   *Drill (Trying to Do It Without the Conversation Topics List)*

CHAPTER 4: THE THREE STEPS OF THE CONVERSATION FRAMEWORK

Students' Conversation	Adult Prompts
Walsh: Have you seen *My Little Pony*, the new one – it's awesome. Pearce: I don't watch it, but I know a lot of people that do. Walsh: It's funny. Walsh: Have you heard of it?	
	Mrs. Kerry: Okay, we're on the topic of *My Little Pony*. Figure out how to include me in the conversation.
Henry: Do you like ponies?	
	Mrs. Kerry: Okay, so you can say "Speaking of ponies …"
Henry: Speaking of ponies, have you ever ridden a horse?	
	Mrs. Kerry: Yes.
Henry: Where?	
	Mrs. Kerry: My mom used to own a horse. I also rode a horse at Oak Mountain and at overnight camp.
Pearce: That's really just like sitting on a horse because you can't gallop.	
	Mrs. Kerry: Okay, pretend that conversation ended. We are on the topic of horses. Horses are under the category of what?
Henry: Animals.	
	Mrs. Kerry: Yes, what else?
Pearce: Pets.	
	Mrs. Kerry: What else?
Pearce: Animals.	
	Mrs. Kerry: Yes, it can be under the category of animals and pets. What other category can it be in?
Henry: Farm animals.	
	Mrs. Kerry: Well, it could be, but that's under the category of animals. Horseback riding is not a TV show, so what category can it be in?
Henry: Hobbies.	
	Mrs. Kerry: Yes.

Considerations

Age of Development

Developmental age is not as important as making sure that the previous steps within the Conversation Framework have been mastered prior to this step. The typical age of development for changing conversation topics begins in elementary school.

Group Size and Setting

If a student has difficulty with bridging the topic, the skill should be addressed in an individual or small-group setting. Group size and background noise matter. It is important that the group size reflects the needs of each individual. Start with the setting that would be the easiest for your student until she masters bridging the topic in that setting. Then work on the skill in more challenging settings.

Just because somebody has demonstrated proficiency in changing conversation topics in one setting with one peer does not mean that he has mastered changing conversation topics in other settings and with others. Practicing conversation in various situations will help the student to generalize skills. Refer to the list of typical group sizes and settings for conversation on pages 17-19 to identify the various places where changing conversation topics might be taught and practiced.

Hesitation Time

Just as with generating stories, questions, and comments, the skill of bridging the topic must be developed to the point that it can be done very rapidly – within 0-2 seconds. If a person takes 10 seconds to generate a related conversation topic to bridge the conversation or takes 10 seconds to determine how to get from one category to another category smoothly, she will most likely be left out of the conversation.

Because individuals with ASD often have difficulty using context to understand social interactions (Vermeulen, 2012), it is imperative to practice conversation in real-life conversation settings. With direct instruction, repeated practice, and positive experience, individuals with ASD can learn to actively participate in back-and-forth conversations that flow naturally.

CHAPTER 5
ASSESSMENTS FOR THE CONVERSATION FRAMEWORK

MEASURING ABILITY AND PROGRESS

Assessments are necessary in order to establish a baseline – the level of a behavior or skill prior to intervention. A baseline should be established before starting intervention and should include detailed information related to a student's ability and challenges. Assessments should be completed for each step of the Conversation Framework.

In addition, continued assessments allow us to track progress over time and to check how effective we are with our teaching. If the student is not progressing, either he is not working on what he needs to or the way we are teaching is not working for him.

Mastery of each skill has been achieved when the student is able to repeatedly and correctly perform a given skill that is being measured in the setting and format. Table 5.1 lists sample target areas and corresponding mastery criteria. Criteria for mastery should represent the needs of your student and direction of your goals. Thus, every individual will have individualized criteria for mastery that change over time. Professional and clinical judgment should guide the criteria.

Table 5.1
Sample Target Areas and Corresponding Criteria for Mastery

Target Area	Criteria for Mastery
Frequency	• Number of times skill was used within a period of time (e.g., 2 comments in 10-minute conversation)
Group Size	• 1 peer or adult • 2 peers • 3 - 5 peers • 6 - 8 peers • 8+ peers
Setting	• Without background noise • With background noise (constant) • With background noise (changing) • Unstructured setting (hallway transition, recess, lunch) • Structured setting (classroom) • Sitting • Standing
Hesitation Time	• 0 - 2 seconds • 2+ seconds • Exact amount of time elapsed
Percentage	• 100% • 90% • 85% • 80% • 75% • 5 out of 5 conversations • 4 out of 5 conversations • 3 out of 5 conversations • 5 out of 5 opportunities • 4 out of 5 opportunities • 3 out of 5 opportunities

Several assessment tools have been included in this chapter for each conversation step to help you measure your student's abilities. The assessment tools measure individual ability. They follow the Conversation Framework; however, please do not allow the assessments to interfere with your clinical judgment. The score on an assessment measure is just one indicator of a skill or area of need. Your instinct and observations beyond the results of an assessment tool are also helpful guides for recognizing student needs and planning teaching strategies.

The assessment tools are not intended to provide comprehensive testing of skills from Step 1 to Step 3 for all students. Only conduct the assessments in the area(s) where you suspect your student is having difficulties. Assessments are intended to identify a starting point in the Conversation Framework. Table 5.2 provides an overview of assessments for each step of the Conversation Framework.

CHAPTER 5: ASSESSMENTS FOR THE CONVERSATION FRAMEWORK

Table 5.2
Overview of Assessments for Each Step in the Conversation Framework

Conversation Step	Name of Assessment
Identifying the Topic	Assessment for Identifying the Topic (4 - 11 Years) Assessment for Identifying the Topic (12 Years - Adult) Assessment for Girls Conversation (12 Years - Adult) Assessment for Implied Emotions (5 Years - 12 Years) Assessment for Implied Emotions (12 Years - Adult) Assessment for Inferred Meaning (12 Years - Adult) Assessment for Recognizing Idioms and Sarcasm (7 Years - Adult)
Balancing the Conversation	Tally Mark Chart (Two People) Tally Mark Chart (Three People) Tally Mark Chart (Four People) Tally Mark Chart (Five People) Tally Mark Chart (Six People) Tally Mark Chart (Seven People) Tally Mark Chart (Eight People)
Asking Questions	Topics for Starting a Conversation With School-Age People You Do Not Know Topics For Starting a Conversation With Adults You Do Not Know Assessment for Questions to Start a Conversation With People You Know Assessment for Follow-Up Questions – Prompted Assessment for Follow-Up Questions – Unprompted Assessment for Reciprocal Questions – Prompted Assessment for Reciprocal Questions – Unprompted
Telling Stories	Assessment for Sequential Story Assessment for Informational Story Assessment for Emotional Story Assessment for Story to Start Conversation Assessment for Related Story
Making Comments	Assessment for Empathetic Comments Assessment for Response Comments
Bridging Topics	Assessment for Bridging Topics

IDENTIFYING THE TOPIC

"Identifying the Topic" is the first step of the Conversation Framework because we must first listen to a conversation and identify the topic before we can ask relevant questions, tell related stories, or make appropriate comments – the other major components of participating in a conversation. Identifying the topic focuses on what is being said. It includes the ability to recognize the overall theme or subject of the conversation as it emerges from the details of a conversation.

The following assessments measure a student's ability to identify the topic. In educational settings, identifying the topic is sometimes referred to as "stating the main idea," a skill that is frequently required for academic subject areas, such as reading and language arts. Since most conversations are verbal (sign language may be used for conversation), identifying the topic is sometimes addressed under the category of listening comprehension.

Two separate areas are required to correctly identify the topic: (a) identifying the overall topic, theme, or subject; and (b) identifying the weight of the conversation.

If you are working with a high-functioning student, consider administering Assessment for Identifying the Topic (12 Years – Adult) or Assessment for Girl Conversation (12 Years – Adult), even if the student is younger than the age requirements. Please use professional judgment to decide if those assessments are appropriate for the student.

Assessment for Identifying the Topic (4 – 11 Years)
Parts One, Two, and Three

Directions: Prior to administering this assessment, ensure the student understands the word *topic* and circle Y (Yes) or N (No). If needed, please explain the concept of a "topic" (see Appendix E).

Depending on the student's needs, the Conversation Topics List (Appendices C and D) may or may not be used as a visual support. Note on the assessment when the Conversation Topics List is used. Using this visual support makes identifying the topic easier, but it is important to gradually remove it to ensure that the student can engage in a conversation without the visual support available. Part Three is designed to be combined with the Conversation Topics List; however, use professional judgment if the student needs the Conversation Topics List in other sections. If the student is working on identifying the topic with background noise, intentional background noise should be used. Circle Y (Yes) or N (No) in the appropriate row at the bottom of the assessment depending on whether or not intentional background noise was used.

The items on the assessments are read aloud because most conversation is spoken. Read the bold sentence(s) out loud at a regular talking speed. Do not slow down the bold sentence(s) because this may make it easier for the student to identify the topic. Allowable prompts are included in each assessment.

Read the items in bold one at a time. After reading each item in Part One, ask the student to state the main topic and circle Y (Yes) or N (No) in the appropriate column. The student should be able to identify the idea in 2 seconds or less. This is important to be able to participate actively in a conversation and not be "left behind" as the other conversation partners move on. Please mark the student's hesitation time in seconds in the space provided. Finally, if the student correctly identifies the topic, follow up by asking the student to describe the weight of the conversation and note the response in the final column. If the student does not understand the concept of the "weight" of the conversation, please use the visual sup-

CHAPTER 5: ASSESSMENTS FOR THE CONVERSATION FRAMEWORK

port for the weight of a conversation (see Appendix G). Students may describe the conversation as Light (L), Medium (M), or Heavy (H), or as Joking (J) or Serious (S), depending on which is most appropriate developmentally. Circle the student's response for Light (L), Medium (M), or Heavy (H), or as Joking (J) or Serious (S). Then circle Y (Yes) or N (No) to show if the weight the student named was correct.

The directions for Part Two and Part Three are very similar to Part One; however, Part Two and Part Three include a larger section for notes. This section may be used to write the student's specific response, information that may be important for communicating with parents, other teachers, or your student's team. After asking about the general topic, ask, "What is the specific topic?" Circle Y (Yes) or N (No) in the appropriate column, depending on whether or not the student was able to verbalize the topic. Continue completing Part Two by recording the student's hesitation time in seconds in the space provided and asking for the weight of the conversation. Note the response in the final column as Light (L), Medium (M), or Heavy (H), or as Joking (J) or Serious (S), depending on which is most appropriate developmentally.

Part One measures the student's ability to identify general topics. Part Two measures the student's ability to identify both general and specific topics. These assessments should be completed in sequential order unless the student scores poorly on Part One and Part Two is not needed. Part Three should only be completed if the student scored poorly on Part One or Two. Part Three allows the use of a copy of the Conversation Topics List (see Appendices C or D). If you use a laminated copy of the Conversation Topics, ask the student to tell you all the topics that it may be or ask him to use a dry-erase marker to mark each topic that might be related to the topic that you say aloud. Record correct and incorrect topics by using tally marks or writing the exact wording of the conversation topic that is stated by the student.

Part One – Identifying the General Topic

Allowable Prompts: *"What is the topic?" "What is the general topic?" "What is the whole thing about?" "A topic is what someone is talking about." "A topic is what the whole thing is about." "Look at the Conversation Topics List." "Use a pen/dry erase marker to mark all the topics that it could be."*			
Does the student understand the word topic?		Y N	
Statement	**Correct Topic? (Y or N)**	**Hesitation Time in Seconds**	**Weight**
1. I went to the beach and found some seashells. What is the topic? General topic: vacation, beach, or things that I did at beach Incorrect response: "I don't know," repeating the entire paragraph, "You were talking too fast," "I got distracted," "I couldn't hear you," seashells Did you have to repeat the bold sentence(s)? How many times? _____	Y N		L M H J S Y N

TALK WITH ME

Statement	Correct Topic? (Y or N)	Hesitation Time in Seconds	Weight
2. My brother went to see Alabama-LSU football game on Saturday. What is the topic? General topic: football, weekend, sports Incorrect response: "I don't know," repeating the entire paragraph, "You were talking too fast," "I got distracted," "I couldn't hear you" Did you have to repeat the bold sentence(s)? Y N If you answered yes, how many times? _____	Y N		L M H J S Y N
3. I've been wanting to take my kids to the water park. What is the topic? General topic: water park, family Incorrect response: "I don't know," repeating the entire paragraph, "You were talking too fast," "I got distracted," "I couldn't hear you" Did you have to repeat the bold sentence(s)? Y N If you answered yes, how many times? _____	Y N		L M H J S Y N
4. I saw *Cloudy With a Chance of Meatballs 2* when it came out in the theater. What is the topic? General topic: movies Incorrect response: "I don't know," repeating the entire paragraph, "You were talking too fast," "I got distracted," "I couldn't hear you" Did you have to repeat the bold sentence(s)? Y N If you answered yes, how many times? _____	Y N		L M H J S Y N
5. Last time I went fishing with my dad, we caught two bass. What is the topic? General topic: fishing, family Incorrect response: "I don't know," repeating the entire paragraph, "You were talking too fast," "I got distracted," "I couldn't hear you," "I don't know what bass is," bass Did you have to repeat the bold sentence(s)? Y N If you answered yes, how many times? _____	Y N		L M H J S Y N
During the assessment, did the student use the Conversation Topics List as a visual support?		Y N	
During the assessment, was there intentional background noise?		Y N	

CHAPTER 5: ASSESSMENTS FOR THE CONVERSATION FRAMEWORK

Part Two – Identifying the General and Specific Topic

Allowable Prompts: *"What is the topic?" "What is the general topic?" "What is the specific topic?" "What is the whole thing about?" "A topic is what someone is talking about." "A topic is what the whole thing is about." "Look at the Conversation Topics List." "Use a pen/dry erase marker to mark all the topics that it could be."*

Does the student understand the word topic?		Y N	
Statement	**Correct Topic? (Y or N)**	**Hesitation Time in Seconds**	**Weight**
1. **I didn't want to come back to school. Over the weekend, I went to my grandparents' house with my sister. When we were there, we played on the Internet, went to a movie, and played outside. What is the general topic? What is the specific topic?** General topic: weekend, family, people/lives, vacation Specific topic: grandparents' house, activities at grandparents (internet, movie, AND played outside) Incorrect response: "I don't know," repeating the entire paragraph, "You were talking too fast," "I got distracted," "I couldn't hear you," stayed there for a long time, played games, didn't want to go to school, school, naming only one activity (internet, movie, OR played outside) Did you have to repeat the bold sentence(s)? Y N If you answered yes, how many times? _____	General Y N Specific Y N		L M H J S Y N
NOTES			
2. **The other day my school went to the zoo. We saw the tigers, elephants, and monkeys. My favorite was the train ride. I'm ready to go back again. What is the general topic? What is the specific topic?** General topic: people/lives, hobbies/interests, zoo, field trip Specific topic: activities at the zoo (tigers, elephants, monkeys, AND train ride) Incorrect response: "I don't know," repeating the entire paragraph, "You were talking too fast," "I got distracted," "I couldn't hear you," school, naming only one activity (tigers, elephants, monkeys, OR train ride) Did you have to repeat the bold sentence(s)? Y N If you answered yes, how many times? _____	General Y N Specific Y N		L M H J S Y N
NOTES			

TALK WITH ME

Statement	Correct Topic? (Y or N)	Hesitation Time in Seconds	Weight
3. I cannot wait to go to the beach this summer. I like swimming in the gulf and the pool. I also like lying in the sun. What is the general topic? What is the specific topic? General topic: vacations, holidays Specific topic: beach, summer, going to the beach Incorrect response: "I don't know," repeating the entire paragraph, "You were talking too fast," "I got distracted," "I couldn't hear you," swimming Did you have to repeat the bold sentence(s)? Y N If you answered yes, how many times? _____	General Y N Specific Y N		L M H J S Y N
NOTES			
4. My family and I went to Disney World for the Fourth of July. We watched the fireworks over Cinderella's castle and rode all of the rides in the park. It was so much fun. What is the general topic? What is the specific topic? General topic: vacation Specific topic: Activities at Disney World (watched fireworks AND rode rides), Fourth of July Incorrect response: "I don't know," repeating the entire paragraph, "You were talking too fast," "I got distracted," "I couldn't hear you," family Did you have to repeat the bold sentence(s)? Y N If you answered yes, how many times? _____	General Y N Specific Y N		L M H J S Y N
NOTES			

CHAPTER 5: ASSESSMENTS FOR THE CONVERSATION FRAMEWORK

Statement	Correct Topic? (Y or N)	Hesitation Time in Seconds	Weight
5. My brothers and I went to see *Seventh Son* because my parents were in a meeting, but in the middle of it, my little brother got sick. We had to leave the movie after only 20 minutes. What is the general topic? What is the specific topic? General topic: movie Specific topic: *Seventh Son*, leaving early because sick brother Incorrect response: "I don't know," repeating the entire paragraph, "You were talking too fast," "I got distracted," "I couldn't hear you," Seven brothers, parents at meeting Did you have to repeat the bold sentence(s)? Y N If you answered yes, how many times? _____	General Y N Specific Y N		L M H J S Y N
NOTES			
During the assessment, did the student use the Conversation Topics List as a visual support?		Y N	
During the assessment, was there intentional background noise?		Y N	

Part Three – Identifying the General Topic Using the Conversation Topics List**
(Appendices C or D)

**Only do this if the student scored poorly on Part One and/or Two.

Allowable Prompts: *"What is the topic?" "What is the general topic?" "What is the whole thing about?" "A topic is what someone is talking about." "A topic is what the whole thing is about." "Look at the Conversation Topics List." "Use a pen/dry erase marker to mark all the topics that it could be under."*			
Does the student understand the word topic?	Y N		
Identifying the General Topic	**Number of Correct Topics**	**Number of Incorrect Topics**	**Hesitation Time in Seconds**
1. I went to the high school football game on Friday night. What topics can that be under? Name all of the topics that it could be. General topics: people/lives, school, hobbies & interests, weekend, sports, family Incorrect response: "I don't know," repeating the entire paragraph, "You were talking too fast," "I got distracted," "I couldn't hear you," topics from the Conversation Topics List that do not match Did you have to repeat the bold sentence(s)? Y N If you answered yes, how many times? _____			
NOTES			
2. I can't believe we got snowed in and missed school. What topics can that be under? Name all of the topics that it could be. General topics: people/lives, school, current events, news, weather, family, weird things Incorrect response: "I don't know," repeating the entire paragraph, "You were talking too fast," "I got distracted," "I couldn't hear you," topics from the Conversation Topics List that do not match Did you have to repeat the bold sentence(s)? Y N If you answered yes, how many times? _____			
NOTES			

CHAPTER 5: ASSESSMENTS FOR THE CONVERSATION FRAMEWORK

3. I remember last winter when my brother jumped into a freezing cold pool. What topics can that be under? Name all of the topics that it could be. General topics: people/lives, hobbies/interests, weather, family, weird things Incorrect response: "I don't know," repeating the entire paragraph, "You were talking too fast," "I got distracted," "I couldn't hear you," topics from the Conversation Topics List that do not match Did you have to repeat the bold sentence(s)? Y N If you answered yes, how many times? _____			
NOTES			
4. I have a difficult project that is due in one week. What topics can that be under? Name all of the topics that it could be. General topics: people/lives, school, emotions Incorrect response: "I don't know," repeating the entire paragraph, "You were talking too fast," "I got distracted," "I couldn't hear you," topics from the Conversation Topics List that do not match Did you have to repeat the bold sentence(s)? Y N If you answered yes, how many times? _____			
NOTES			
5. Today after school, I am buying a new video game. What topics can that be under? Name all of the topics that it could be. General topics: people/lives, hobbies/interests, electronics, family Incorrect response: "I don't know," repeating the entire paragraph, "You were talking too fast," "I got distracted," "I couldn't hear you," topics from the Conversation Topics List that do not match Did you have to repeat the bold sentence(s)? Y N If you answered yes, how many times? _____			
NOTES			
During the assessment, did the student use the Conversation Topics List as a visual support?		(Y)	N
During the assessment, was there intentional background noise?		Y	N

Assessment for Identifying the Topic (12 Years – Adult)

Directions: If the student is high-functioning, consider using this assessment to measure the ability to identify the topic, regardless of the age requirements listed. Please use professional judgment to decide if this assessment is appropriate.

Prior to administering this assessment, ensure the student understands the word *topic* and circle Y (Yes) or N (No). If needed, please explain the concept of a "topic" (see Appendix E). This assessment measures the student's ability to state the general and specific topic. If needed, please reference the visual support for teaching the difference between general and specific topics in Appendix F.

Read the items in bold one at a time, each time asking, "What is the topic?" If needed, use a visual to explain the concept of "topic" to support the student in responding to the assessment questions. Depending on the student's needs, the Conversation Topics List may or may not be used as a visual support. Note on the assessment when the Conversation Topics List is used. Using this visual support makes identifying the topic easier, but it is important to gradually remove it to ensure that the student can engage in a conversation without the visual support available. If the student is working on identifying the topic with background noise, intentional background noise should be used. Circle Y (Yes) or N (No) in the appropriate row at the bottom of the assessment depending on whether or not intentional background noise was used.

The items on the assessments are read aloud because most conversation is spoken. Read the bold sentence(s) at a regular talking speed. Do not slow down the bold sentence(s) because this may make it easier for the student to identify the topic. Allowable prompts at the top of the assessment.

After reading each item, ask the student to state the topic and circle Y (Yes) or N (No) in the appropriate column. The general topics match topics on the Conversation Topics List in Appendices C and D. The student should be able to identify the topic in 2 seconds or less. This is important to be able to participate actively in a conversation and not be "left behind" as the other conversation partners move on. Please mark the student's total hesitation time in seconds in the space provided. After asking about the general topic, ask, "What is the specific topic?" Circle Y (Yes) or N (No) in the appropriate column, depending on whether or not the student was able to verbalize the specific topic. Again, mark the student's total hesitation time in seconds in the space provided. Finally, if the student correctly identifies the topic, follow up by asking the student to describe the weight of the conversation and note the response in the final column. If the student does not understand the concept of the "weight" of the conversation, please use the visual support for the weight of a conversation (see Appendix G). Students may describe the conversation as Light (L), Medium (M), or Heavy (H), or as Joking (J) or Serious (S), depending on which is most appropriate developmentally. Circle the student's response for Light (L), Medium (M), or Heavy (H), or as Joking (J) or Serious (S). Then circle Y (Yes) or N (No) to show if the weight the student named was correct.

CHAPTER 5: ASSESSMENTS FOR THE CONVERSATION FRAMEWORK

Allowable Prompts: *"What is the topic?" "What is the general topic?" "What is the specific topic?" "What is the whole thing about?" "A topic is what someone is talking about." "A topic is what the whole thing is about."*			
Does the student understand the word topic?		Y N	
Statement	**Correct Topic? (Y or N)**	**Hesitation Time in Seconds**	**Weight**
1. I think Ben Affleck will do a great job as Batman. He'll definitely do better than George Clooney did in that role. However, my all-time favorite Batman was Christian Bale. **What is the topic? What is the specific topic?**	General Y N		L M H J S Y N
General topic: movies, hobbies/interests			
Specific topic: actors, Batman			
Incorrect response: "I don't know," repeating the entire paragraph, "You were talking too fast," "I got distracted," "I couldn't hear you," George Clooney	Specific Y N		
Did you have to repeat the bold sentence(s)? Y N			
If you answered yes, how many times? _____			
NOTES			
2. I cannot believe the basketball game last night. The teams went into overtime, and it was a real nail-biter. I really wanted the Nets to win. They seriously choked. **What is the topic? What is the specific topic?**	General Y N		L M H J S Y N
General topic: sports/basketball, last night, hobbies/interests, news			
Specific topic: Nets team			
Incorrect response: "I don't know," repeating the entire paragraph, "You were talking too fast," "I got distracted," "I couldn't hear you"	Specific Y N		
Did you have to repeat the bold sentence(s)? Y N			
If you answered yes, how many times? _____			
NOTES			

TALK WITH ME

Statement	Correct Topic? (Y or N)	Hesitation Time in Seconds	Weight
3. I met this guy who wants to start beehives. I looked online and found out that the cost of the beehive is around $4,000, and the queen bee is pretty expensive, too. I wonder if you can get your money back if the queen bee dies. **What is the topic? What is the specific topic?** General topic: jobs, people/lives, hobbies/interests Specific topic: starting beehives, beehives Incorrect response: "I don't know," repeating the entire paragraph, "You were talking too fast," "I got distracted," "I couldn't hear you" Did you have to repeat the bold sentence(s)? Y N If you answered yes, how many times? _____	General Y N Specific Y N		L M H J S Y N
NOTES			
4. I didn't get to see the official replay, but those types of things happen. Some people make bad calls or calls that I wouldn't agree with. Either way, the game ended the way it should have. **What is the topic? What is the specific topic?** General topic: sports, weekends, games Specific topic: fairness of a game, or specific game/sport (e.g. football, baseball, basketball) Incorrect response: "I don't know," repeating the entire paragraph, "You were talking too fast," "I got distracted," "I couldn't hear you" Did you have to repeat the bold sentence(s)? Y N If you answered yes, how many times? _____	General Y N Specific Y N		L M H J S Y N
NOTES			

CHAPTER 5: ASSESSMENTS FOR THE CONVERSATION FRAMEWORK

Statement	Correct Topic? (Y or N)	Hesitation Time in Seconds	Weight
5. I know you were in New Orleans. I can't believe what happened out there with the hurricanes. I don't think I've seen the rebuilding of a city quite like that before. They've really done a great job rebuilding everything and bringing the town back together in the wake of a tragedy. What is the topic? What is the specific topic? General topic: news, weather, current events, people/lives Specific topic: rebuilding New Orleans, hurricanes, New Orleans Did you have to repeat the bold sentence(s)? Y N If you answered yes, how many times? _____	General Y N Specific Y N		L M H J S Y N
NOTES			
6. I don't think I've ever heard the roar of the crowd that loud. It reminded me of the Alabama-Florida game a few years back where the crowd went wild. Being there was absolutely incredible. I was lucky enough to have gotten tickets. What is the topic? What is the specific topic? General topic: sports, weekends; Specific topic: people/lives, being at a game, football Incorrect response: "I don't know," repeating the entire paragraph, "You were talking too fast," "I got distracted," "I couldn't hear you," getting tickets, news Did you have to repeat the bold sentence(s)? Y N If you answered yes, how many times? _____	General Y N Specific Y N		L M H J S Y N
NOTES			

TALK WITH ME

Statement	Correct Topic? (Y or N)	Hesitation Time in Seconds	Weight
7. My dad's side of the family lives here. My mom's side of the family lives in Minnesota. We went up there last Christmas when it was snowing. It was pretty fun seeing everyone because I haven't been there for a while. Now that I live in Alabama, we really don't have season changes like they do in Minnesota. What is the topic? What is the specific topic? General topic: people/lives, family, places, weather Specific topic: season changes, snow, vacations, or Christmas Incorrect response: "I don't know," repeating the entire paragraph, "You were talking too fast," "I got distracted," "I couldn't hear you" Did you have to repeat the bold sentence(s)? Y N If you answered yes, how many times? _____	General Y N Specific Y N		L M H J S Y N
NOTES			
8. No, I don't play paintball. If I wanted to be shot at, I'd join the army. I just prefer playing it on video games. I did go last summer with a group of guys, but the welts did not go away for a week. Who wants to do that to themselves and call that fun? What is the topic? What is the specific topic? General topic: people/lives, hobbies/interests, places, sports Specific topic: paintball, summer, video games Incorrect response: "I don't know," repeating the entire paragraph, "You were talking too fast," "I got distracted," "I couldn't hear you," weekend Did you have to repeat the bold sentence(s)? Y N If you answered yes, how many times? _____	General Y N Specific Y N		L M H J S Y N
NOTES			

CHAPTER 5: ASSESSMENTS FOR THE CONVERSATION FRAMEWORK

Statement	Correct Topic? (Y or N)	Hesitation Time in Seconds	Weight
9. I was watching this documentary comparing the British long sword to the katana (kuh-tah-nah). They were both swords made using the same material and the same method, but the katana could stab or slice through armor so much better because of the shape of it. What is the topic? What is the specific topic? General topic: hobbies/interests, electronics, TV shows Specific topic: last night, documentaries, history, weapons, swords, katana Incorrect response: "I don't know," repeating the entire paragraph, "You were talking too fast," "I got distracted," "I couldn't hear you" Did you have to repeat the bold sentence(s)? Y N If you answered yes, how many times? _____	General Y N Specific Y N		L M H J S Y N
NOTES			
10. We went to Key West for a wedding. For some reason I could not hear. The doctor said that my Eustachian tubes were backed up. I've never heard of that before. I had to get help with the volume for the slideshow at the rehearsal dinner because I couldn't hear a thing. I couldn't tell if the sound was even on or if it was too loud. What is the topic? What is the specific topic? General topic: people/lives, family, weird things Specific topic: sickness, couldn't hear, hearing, rehearsal dinner Incorrect response: "I don't know," repeating the entire paragraph, "You were talking too fast," "I got distracted," "I couldn't hear you," wedding, Key West Did you have to repeat the bold sentence(s)? Y N If you answered yes, how many times? _____	General Y N Specific Y N		L M H J S Y N
NOTES			

TALK WITH ME

Statement	Correct Topic? (Y or N)	Hesitation Time in Seconds	Weight
11. Just got word that there was an arrest in my neighborhood. Apparently, there was a guy who was celebrating Halloween a few days early walking the neighborhood in full Duck Dynasty attire – definitely a fake beard as a disguise. That seemed to be his cover for breaking into houses. Unbelievable. What is the topic? What is the specific topic? General topic: weird things, current events Specific topic: Halloween, holidays, costumes, Duck Dynasty, break-ins, arrests, burglaries Incorrect response: "I don't know," repeating the entire paragraph, "You were talking too fast," "I got distracted," "I couldn't hear you," Halloween Did you have to repeat the bold sentence(s)? Y N If you answered yes, how many times? _____	General Y N Specific Y N		L M H J S Y N
NOTES			
12. It looked like it was embedded in a video game. It was the most technologically spectacular Super Bowl ever. I don't know that you could top it in terms of the technology used. You know my question is if she lip-synced. Either way, I'm ready for someone to go out there and sing. What is the topic? What is the specific topic? General topic: electronics, sports, weekends Specific topic: Super Bowl halftime show, singer, entertainer, technology Incorrect topics: "I don't know," repeating the entire paragraph, "You were talking too fast," "I got distracted," "I couldn't hear you," video games, game(s), person (too vague) Did you have to repeat the bold sentence(s)? Y N If you answered yes, how many times? _____	General Y N Specific Y N		L M H J S Y N
NOTES			
During the assessment, did the student use the Conversation Topics List as a visual support?	Y N		
During the assessment, was there intentional background noise?	Y N		

CHAPTER 5: ASSESSMENTS FOR THE CONVERSATION FRAMEWORK

Assessment for Girl Conversation (12 Years – Adult)

Directions: If the student is high-functioning, consider using this assessment to measure the ability to identify the topic ,regardless of the age requirements listed. Please use professional judgment to decide if this assessment is appropriate for the student.

The items on the assessments are read aloud because most conversation is spoken. Read the bold sentence(s) at a regular talking speed. Do not slow down the bold sentence(s) because this may make it easier for the student to identify the topic. Allowable prompts at the top of the assessment.

Read the items in bold one at a time, each time asking, "What is the topic?" After reading each item, ask the student to state the topic and circle Y (Yes) or N (No) in the appropriate column. The student should be able to identify the topic in 2 seconds or less. This is important to be able to participate actively in a conversation and not be "left behind" as the other conversation partners move on. Please mark the student's total hesitation time in seconds in the space provided. Even though acceptable responses are listed as main topic and emotion, many girls recognize the emotion as the main topic. Ask the student to label the emotion unless she labeled the emotion as part of the topic. Ask, "Why would he/she be feeling that emotion?" Circle Y (Yes) or N (No) to identify if the correct emotion was identified. Also, circle Y (Yes) or N (No) if the student was able to provide appropriate justification as to why the person would be feeling the emotion stated.

If the student has difficulty identifying emotion words, consider using the Emotion List as a visual support (see Appendix H). Circle Y (Yes) or N (No) in the appropriate row at the bottom of the assessment depending on whether or not the Emotion List was used.

Finally, follow up by asking the student to describe the weight of the conversation and note the response in the final column. If the student does not understand the concept of the "weight" of the conversation, use the visual support for the weight of a conversation (see Appendix G). Students may describe the conversation as Light (L), Medium (M), or Heavy (H), or as Joking (J) or Serious (S), depending on which is most appropriate developmentally. Circle the student's response for Light (L), Medium (M), or Heavy (H), or as Joking (J) or Serious (S). Then circle Y (Yes) or N (No) to show if the weight the student named was correct.

TALK WITH ME

Allowable prompts: *"What's the topic?" "What's the emotion?" "What emotion is that?" "Take a guess." "What is my/his/her emotion?" "The emotion would be what the person is feeling." "Give me an emotion word." "Why would I/he/she be feeling that emotion?"*

Statement	Correct Topic? (Y or N)	Hesitation Time in Seconds	Correct Emotion and Justification? (Y or N)	Weight
1. Did you see what she was wearing? I cannot believe how short her skirt is. That's so insane that she does not get in trouble for that. What is the topic? What is my emotion (if an emotion was not labeled already)? Why would I be feeling that emotion? Main topic: bad choice of skirt, how she wore a really short skirt, dress code Emotion: disgust, confused, shocked (bad) Incorrect Responses: "I don't know," repeating the entire paragraph, "You were talking too fast," "I got distracted," "I couldn't hear you," fashion, person being mean to a girl Did you have to repeat the bold sentence(s)? Y N If you answered yes, how many times? _____ Number of Correct Emotions Named: _____	Y N		Correct Emotion? Y N Correct Justification? Y N	L M H J S Y N
NOTES				
2. I wouldn't want to go against her on anything. She's such a gossip. I'd be afraid that she'd start talking about me. The other day she was talking about Jessica – did you hear her talking about that? What is the topic? What is my emotion (if an emotion was not labeled already)? Why would I be feeling that emotion? Main topic: gossiping about someone gossiping Emotion: worried, suspicious, self-conscious Incorrect Responses: "I don't know," repeating the entire paragraph, "You were talking too fast," "I got distracted," "I couldn't hear you," friends Did you have to repeat the bold sentence(s)? Y N If you answered yes, how many times? _____ Number of Correct Emotions Named: _____	Y N		Correct Emotion? Y N Correct Justification? Y N	L M H J S Y N
NOTES				

CHAPTER 5: ASSESSMENTS FOR THE CONVERSATION FRAMEWORK

Statement	Correct Topic? (Y or N)	Hesitation Time in Seconds	Correct Emotion and Justification? (Y or N)	Weight
3. I didn't make the tennis team this year. I was on the tennis team last year, but I don't know what happened this time. **What is the topic? What is my emotion (if an emotion was not labeled already)? Why would I be feeling that emotion?** Main topic: disappointment, not making the tennis team Emotion: disappointed, sad, embarrassed, shocked (bad), surprised (bad) Incorrect Responses: "I don't know," repeating the entire paragraph, "You were talking too fast," "I got distracted," "I couldn't hear you," sports, not practicing, needing to try harder, practice makes perfect Did you have to repeat the bold sentence(s)? Y N If you answered yes, how many times? _____ Number of Correct Emotions Named: _____	Y N		Correct Emotion? Y N Correct Justification? Y N	L M H J S Y N
NOTES				
4. I'm so tired of my sister hogging the bathroom. She takes waaaayyyy too long. She is so inconsiderate. I have to get ready too. **What is the topic? What is my emotion (if an emotion was not labeled already)? Why would I be feeling that emotion?** Main topic: sister in bathroom, sister taking too long Emotion: annoyed, angry, frustrated, impatient, irritated Incorrect Responses: "I don't know," repeating the entire paragraph, "You were talking too fast," "I got distracted," "I couldn't hear you," sister (too vague) Did you have to repeat the bold sentence(s)? Y N If you answered yes, how many times? _____ Number of Correct Emotions Named: _____	Y N		Correct Emotion? Y N Correct Justification? Y N	L M H J S Y N
NOTES				

TALK WITH ME

Statement	Correct Topic? (Y or N)	Hesitation Time in Seconds	Correct Emotion and Justification? (Y or N)	Weight
5. I really wanted these new shoes, but my mom said I already have too many shoes. She won't even let me get a job in the summer, so I could make money to be able to buy them for myself. What is the topic? What is my emotion (if an emotion was not labeled already)? Why would I be feeling that emotion? Main topic: mom not giving her what she wanted, wanting new shoes Emotion: frustration, disappointed, confused (why she isn't allowed to get a job) Incorrect Responses: "I don't know," repeating the entire paragraph, "You were talking too fast," "I got distracted," "I couldn't hear you," getting a job Did you have to repeat the bold sentence(s)? Y N If you answered yes, how many times? _____ Number of Correct Emotions Named: _____	Y N		Correct Emotion? Y N Correct Justification? Y N	L M H J S Y N
NOTES				
6. Are you kidding me! This is the third time they have gotten in front of me in line and no one is doing anything about it. What is the topic? What is my emotion (if an emotion was not labeled already)? Why would I be feeling that emotion? Main topic: someone cutting in line Emotion: frustration, angry Incorrect Responses: "I don't know," repeating the entire paragraph, "You were talking too fast," "I got distracted," "I couldn't hear you," non-related bad things to happen when adults don't do anything to help Did you have to repeat the bold sentence(s)? Y N If you answered yes, how many times? _____ Number of Correct Emotions Named: _____	Y N		Correct Emotion? Y N Correct Justification? Y N	L M H J S Y N
NOTES				

CHAPTER 5: ASSESSMENTS FOR THE CONVERSATION FRAMEWORK

Statement	Correct Topic? (Y or N)	Hesitation Time in Seconds	Correct Emotion and Justification? (Y or N)	Weight
7. I love kittens. Look at how cute this picture is. My mom won't let me have one. We got into a fight about it last night because she doesn't think that I will take care of it. What is the topic? What is my emotion (if an emotion was not labeled already)? Why would I be feeling that emotion? Main topic: mom won't let me have a kitten Emotion: frustration, sad, disappointment, surprised (bad) Incorrect Responses: "I don't know," repeating the entire paragraph, "You were talking too fast," "I got distracted," "I couldn't hear you," excited, happy, cute kittens, kittens, Did you have to repeat the bold sentence(s)? Y N If you answered yes, how many times? _____ Number of Correct Emotions Named: _____	Y N		Correct Emotion? Y N Correct Justification? Y N	L M H J S Y N
NOTES				
8. Did you see the new guy? He's hot. Don't tell anyone I said that. What is the topic? What is my emotion (if an emotion was not labeled already)? Why would I be feeling that emotion? Main topic: crush on new guy, keeping secrets Emotion: worried (that he'll/she'll tell someone), excited, happy Incorrect Responses: "I don't know," repeating the entire paragraph, "You were talking too fast," "I got distracted," "I couldn't hear you," Did you have to repeat the bold sentence(s)? Y N If you answered yes, how many times? _____ Number of Correct Emotions Named: _____	Y N		Correct Emotion? Y N Correct Justification? Y N	L M H J S Y N
NOTES				

TALK WITH ME

Statement	Correct Topic? (Y or N)	Hesitation Time in Seconds	Correct Emotion and Justification? (Y or N)	Weight
9. My little sister likes to steal all of my favorite outfits. She never asks if she can borrow them. She always takes them without asking. What is the topic? What is my emotion (if an emotion was not labeled already)? Why would I be feeling that emotion? Main topic: taking things without asking, sister taking stuff/clothes Emotion: mad, frustrated, angry Incorrect Responses: "I don't know," repeating the entire paragraph, "You were talking too fast," "I got distracted," "I couldn't hear you" Did you have to repeat the bold sentence(s)? Y N If you answered yes, how many times? _____ Number of Correct Emotions Named: _____	Y N		Correct Emotion? Y N Correct Justification? Y N	L M H J S Y N
NOTES				
10. I really wanted to go see a movie with my friends this Friday, but my mom won't let me go. She said I can't go because I didn't clean my room. What is the topic? What is my emotion (if an emotion was not labeled already)? Why would I be feeling that emotion? Main topic: wanting to go to the movies, mom won't let me go to the movies Emotion: frustrated, disappointed, angry, upset Incorrect Responses: "I don't know," repeating the entire paragraph, "You were talking too fast," "I got distracted," "I couldn't hear you," cleaning room Did you have to repeat the bold sentence(s)? Y N If you answered yes, how many times? _____ Number of Correct Emotions Named: _____	Y N		Correct Emotion? Y N Correct Justification? Y N	L M H J S Y N
NOTES				

CHAPTER 5: ASSESSMENTS FOR THE CONVERSATION FRAMEWORK

Statement	Correct Topic? (Y or N)	Hesitation Time in Seconds	Correct Emotion and Justification? (Y or N)	Weight
11. Tommy asked me to the dance this Saturday. I haven't gone to a dance before. I hope he thinks I'm a good dancer. What is the topic? What is my emotion (if an emotion was not labeled already)? Why would I be feeling that emotion? Main topic: school dance, first dance, Tommy invited me to the dance Emotion: hopeful, nervous, excited Incorrect Responses: "I don't know," repeating the entire paragraph, "You were talking too fast," "I got distracted," "I couldn't hear you," good dancer Did you have to repeat the bold sentence(s)? Y N If you answered yes, how many times? _____ Number of Correct Emotions Named: _____	Y N		Correct Emotion? Y N Correct Justification? Y N	L M H J S Y N
NOTES				
During the assessment, did the student use the Conversation Topics List as a visual support?	Y N			
During the assessment, did the student use the Emotion List as a visual support?	Y N			

Assessment for Implied Emotions (5 – 12 Years)

Directions: The items on the assessments are read aloud because most conversation is spoken. Read the bold sentence(s) at a regular talking speed. Do not slow down the bold sentence(s) because this may make it easier for the student to identify the topic. Allowable prompts at the top of the assessment.

After reading each item, ask the student to state the underlying emotion and circle Y (Yes) or N (No) in the appropriate column. Use the allowable prompts if the student does not understand the phrasing of your question about emotions. Circle Y (Yes) or N (No) to show whether the correct emotion was identified. Also, circle Y (Yes) or N (No) if the student was able to provide appropriate justification for why the person would be feeling the emotion stated. If the student gives an acceptable explanation for why an emotion is different from the suggested emotion, consider it a correct response. The student should be able to suggest an emotion in 2 seconds or less. This is important to be able to participate actively in a conversation and not be "left behind" as the other conversation partners move on. Please mark the student's total hesitation time in seconds in the space provided.

If the student has difficulty identifying emotion words, consider using the Emotion List as a visual support (see Appendix H). Circle Y (Yes) or N (No) in the appropriate row at the bottom of the assessment, depending on whether or not the Emotion List was used.

Finally, follow up by asking the student to describe the weight of the conversation and note the response in the final column. If the student does not understand the concept of the "weight" of the conversation, use the visual support for the weight of a conversation (see Appendix G). Students may describe the conversation as Light (L), Medium (M), or Heavy (H), or as Joking (J) or Serious (S), depending on which is most appropriate developmentally. Circle the student's response for Light (L), Medium (M), or Heavy (H), or as Joking (J) or Serious (S). Then circle Y (Yes) or N (No) to show if the weight the student named was correct.

Allowable prompts: *"What's the topic?" "What's the emotion?" "What emotion is that?" "Take a guess." "What is his/her emotion?" "The emotion would be what the person is feeling." "Give me an emotion word." "Why would he/she be feeling that emotion?" "Can you say an emotion?" "What other emotion could that be?"*			
Statement	**Correct Emotion and Justification? (Y or N)**	**Hesitation Time in Seconds**	**Weight**
1. The other day in school, I was in English, and I walked out into the hallway. I was really confused at first because no one was making a sound, and I hadn't ever heard it that quiet. I asked someone what was going on, and they said that someone in the school had died that morning. What is the underlying emotion? Main emotion: sad Did you have to repeat the bold sentence(s)? Y N If you answered yes, how many times? _____	Correct Emotion? Y N Correct Justification? Y N		L M H J S Y N
2. I was at camp one year, and the other counselors found a rattlesnake. Knowing that I have a phobia of snakes, they killed it and pretended to throw it on me. What is the underlying emotion? Main emotion: scared Did you have to repeat the bold sentence(s)? Y N If you answered yes, how many times? _____	Correct Emotion? Y N Correct Justification? Y N		L M H J S Y N
3. I left my iPad there for 1 minute, and now it's gone. I know someone stole it from me! You teachers are supposed to protect me from stuff like that. I hate you idiots! What is the underlying emotion? Main emotion: mad, angry Did you have to repeat the bold sentence(s)? Y N If you answered yes, how many times? _____	Correct Emotion? Y N Correct Justification? Y N		L M H J S Y N

CHAPTER 5: ASSESSMENTS FOR THE CONVERSATION FRAMEWORK

Statement	Correct Emotion and Justification? (Y or N)	Hesitation Time in Seconds	Weight
4. **At practice the other day, my coach told me to go get the camera and film the kickers. While I was on the way to get the camera, another coach told me that I needed to be running with the rest of the offense then took off, and I wasn't sure what to do. If I didn't get the camera, the first coach would be mad at me, but if I got caught not running, the second coach would be mad.** What is the underlying emotion? Main emotion: confused Did you have to repeat the bold sentence(s)? Y N If you answered yes, how many times? _____	Correct Emotion? Y N Correct Justification? Y N		L M H J S Y N
5. **My cat had kittens. They are so cute. We are having so much fun playing with them. I love cats.** What is the underlying emotion? Main emotion: happy Did you have to repeat the bold sentence(s)? Y N If you answered yes, how many times? _____	Correct Emotion? Y N Correct Justification? Y N		L M H J S Y N
During the assessment, did the student use the Emotion List as a visual support?	Y N		

Assessment for Implied Emotions (12 Years – Adult)

Directions: The items on the assessments are read aloud because most conversation is spoken. Read the bold sentence(s) at a regular talking speed. Do not slow down the bold sentence(s) because this may make it easier for the student to identify the topic. Allowable prompts at the top of the assessment.

After reading each item, ask the student to state the underlying emotion and circle Y (Yes) or N (No) in the appropriate column. Use the allowable prompts if the student does not understand the phrasing of your question about emotions. Circle Y (Yes) or N (No) to show whether the correct emotion was identified. Also, circle Y (Yes) or N (No) if the student was able to provide appropriate justification for why the person would be feeling the emotion stated. If the student gives an acceptable explanation for why an emotion is different from the suggested emotion, consider it a correct response. The student should be able to suggest an emotion in 2 seconds or less. This is important to be able to participate actively in a conversation and not be "left behind" as the other conversation partners move on. Please mark the student's total hesitation time in seconds in the space provided.

If the student has difficulty identifying emotion words, consider using the Emotion List as a visual support (see Appendix H). Circle Y (Yes) or N (No) in the appropriate row at the bottom of the assessment depending on whether or not the Emotion List was used.

Finally, follow up by asking the student to describe the weight of the conversation and note the response in the final column. If the student does not understand the concept of the "weight" of the conversation, use the visual support for the weight of a conversation (see Appendix G). Students may describe the conversation as Light (L), Medium (M), or Heavy (H), or as Joking (J) or Serious (S), depending on which is most appropriate developmentally. Circle the student's response for Light (L), Medium (M), or Heavy (H), or as Joking (J) or Serious (S). Then circle Y (Yes) or N (No) to show if the weight the student named was correct.

Allowable prompts: *"What's the topic?" "What's the emotion?" "What emotion is that?" "Take a guess." "What is his/her emotion?" "The emotion would be what the person is feeling." "Give me an emotion word." "Why would he/she be feeling that emotion?" "Can you say an emotion?" "What other emotion could that be?"*

Statement	Correct Emotion and Justification? (Y or N)	Hesitation Time in Seconds	Weight
1. I opened my front door, and my dog ran out before I could stop him. He went straight for the road and got hit by a car. The vet said he probably won't make it. Main emotion: shocked, bad, disbelief, sad Did you have to repeat the bold sentence(s)? Y N If you answered yes, how many times? _____	Correct Emotion? Y N Correct Justification? Y N		L M H J S Y N
2. I wanted to go, but they didn't invite me. I ended up spending the weekend at home by myself. Main emotion: confused, disappointed, hurt, upset, distressed, sad, lonely, frustrated Did you have to repeat the bold sentence(s)? Y N If you answered yes, how many times? _____	Correct Emotion? Y N Correct Justification? Y N		L M H J S Y N
3. I don't know why she always gets to go and I don't. I wish I had a chance to go to that store, too. Main emotion: jealous Did you have to repeat the bold sentence(s)? Y N If you answered yes, how many times? _____	Correct Emotion? Y N Correct Justification? Y N		L M H J S Y N
4. I'm so tired of them complaining. Every time I mention wanting to do anything, they immediately whine about it. Main emotion: annoyed, frustrated Did you have to repeat the bold sentence(s)? Y N If you answered yes, how many times? _____	Correct Emotion? Y N Correct Justification? Y N		L M H J S Y N

CHAPTER 5: ASSESSMENTS FOR THE CONVERSATION FRAMEWORK

Statement	Correct Emotion and Justification? (Y or N)	Hesitation Time in Seconds	Weight
5. I went to the Lego Store. I wanted this really cool house Lego. It even has a garage. It's a two-story Lego house, too. They ran out of them right before I got there. Main emotion: disappointed, sad Did you have to repeat the bold sentence(s)? Y N If you answered yes, how many times? _____	Correct Emotion? Y N Correct Justification? Y N		L M H J S Y N
6. We played really well this past weekend in the soccer tournament. Our coach said it would be hard to play this other team because they were older than us, but we scored the first goal. We lost in overtime, but we played well. Main emotion: confident, proud Did you have to repeat the bold sentence(s)? Y N If you answered yes, how many times? _____	Correct Emotion? Y N Correct Justification? Y N		L M H J S Y N
7. I don't like leaving John home alone. He's too young, and if something happens, he won't be able to contact us. Main emotion: worried Did you have to repeat the bold sentence(s)? Y N If you answered yes, how many times? _____	Correct Emotion? Y N Correct Justification? Y N		L M H J S Y N
8. Did you really do that? Are you sure? Main emotion: doubt, skeptical, shocked, surprised Did you have to repeat the bold sentence(s)? Y N If you answered yes, how many times? _____	Correct Emotion? Y N Correct Justification? Y N		L M H J S Y N
9. I pushed over something at my neighbor's house. It didn't break, but he was pretty upset. I had to go home. Main emotion: guilty Did you have to repeat the bold sentence(s)? Y N If you answered yes, how many times? _____	Correct Emotion? Y N Correct Justification? Y N		L M H J S Y N

Statement	Correct Emotion and Justification? (Y or N)	Hesitation Time in Seconds	Weight
10. There's nothing to do, but I'm fine. I just don't want to talk right now. Main emotion: bored Did you have to repeat the bold sentence(s)? Y N If you answered yes, how many times? _____	Correct Emotion? Y N Correct Justification? Y N		L M H J S Y N
11. Okay?! I'm really not sure what to say here. Main emotion: awkward, uncomfortable, embarrassed, confused Did you have to repeat the bold sentence(s)? Y N If you answered yes, how many times? _____	Correct Emotion? Y N Correct Justification? Y N		L M H J S Y N
During the assessment, did the student use the Emotion List as a visual support?	Y N		

Assessment for Inferred Meaning (12 Years – Adult)

Directions: The items on the assessments are read aloud because most conversation is spoken. Read the bold sentence(s) at a regular talking speed. Do not slow down the bold sentence(s) because this may make it easier for the student to identify the topic. Allowable prompts at the top of the assessment.

After reading each item, ask the student to state the correct meaning by asking, "What is he *really* saying?" Once the student has responded, circle Y (Yes) or N (No) in the appropriate column to identify both if the student was able to determine the correct meaning and if the student stated a literal response. The student should be able to suggest an appropriate meaning in 2 seconds or less. This is important to be able to participate actively in a conversation and not be "left behind" as the other conversation partners move on. Please mark the student's total hesitation time in seconds in the space provided.

Allowable prompts: *"What does that mean?" "Why would they say that?" "Why would they ask that?"*		
Statement	Correct Meaning or Literal Response? (Y or N)	Hesitation Time in Seconds
Ex. I'm hungry. What is he really saying? Response: *He's hungry.* Correct response(s): Please fix something for me to eat; Let's go eat. Incorrect response(s): *Restating the sentence without inferring additional meaning or application, they are hungry. They haven't eaten in a while. Someone is saying they're hungry.* Did you have to repeat the bold sentence(s)? Y N If you answered yes, how many times? _____	Correct Meaning? Y (N) Literal Response? (Y) N	4 seconds

CHAPTER 5: ASSESSMENTS FOR THE CONVERSATION FRAMEWORK

Statement	Correct Meaning or Literal Response? (Y or N)	Hesitation Time in Seconds
1. It's getting late. Isn't it time for your parents to be here? What is he really saying? Response: Correct response(s): It is time for you to leave; I'm ready for you to go. Incorrect response(s): Restating the sentence without inferring additional meaning or application, it's late. Someone is saying it's late, It's getting close to night. Did you have to repeat the bold sentence(s)? Y N If you answered yes, how many times? _____	Correct Meaning? Y N Literal Response? Y N	
2. This luggage is really heavy. What is she really saying? Response: Correct response(s): Help me carry it. Incorrect response(s): Restating the sentence without inferring additional meaning or application. it's heavy, the luggage is heavy, It's hard to carry, It's hard to carry and lift. Did you have to repeat the bold sentence(s)? Y N If you answered yes, how many times? _____	Correct Meaning? Y N Literal Response? Y N	
3. Do you know where my bags went? What is she really saying? Response: Correct response(s): I am wondering if you took them and put them somewhere. Help me look for them. Incorrect response(s): Restating the sentence without inferring additional meaning or application. Someone is looking for the bags, I'm looking for the bags. Where are the bags? Did you have to repeat the bold sentence(s)? Y N If you answered yes, how many times? _____	Correct Meaning? Y N Literal Response? Y N	
4. Have you seen my keys? What is he really saying? Response: Correct response(s): Help me look for them, did you move them? Incorrect response(s): Restating the sentence without inferring additional meaning or application, I'm looking for my keys. Did you have to repeat the bold sentence(s)? Y N If you answered yes, how many times? _____	Correct Meaning? Y N Literal Response? Y N	

Statement	Correct Meaning Or Literal Response? (Y or N)	Hesitation Time in Seconds
5. I guess I can drive for a little while. What is she really saying? Response: Correct response: I will need a break soon, I will need someone else to drive ssoon, I would rather someone else drive. I don't want to drive anymore. Incorrect responses: Restating the sentence without inferring additional meaning or application. I don't need anyone else to drive. I can drive for a little while/short amount of time. Did you have to repeat the bold sentence(s)? How many times?	Correct Meaning? Y N Literal Response? Y N	
6. That trash smells bad. What is he really saying? Response: Correct response: Take the trash out, put it in an air-tight bag where the smell remains contained. Incorrect responses: Restating the sentence without inferring additional meaning or application, the trash stinks. It smells awful. Did you have to repeat the bold sentence(s)? Y N If you answered yes, how many times? _____	Correct Meaning? Y N Literal Response? Y N	
7. Do you have any homework? What are they really saying? Response: Correct response: Do your homework right now, get it out now. I need you to start on it now. Incorrect responses: Restating the sentence without inferring additional meaning or application. I want to know what homework you have. Do you have homework? Did you have to repeat the bold sentence(s)? Y N If you answered yes, how many times? _____	Correct Meaning? Y N Literal Response? Y N	
8. Are you hungry? What is she really saying? Response: Correct response: I want to eat, I'm hungry, I'm ready to eat. Incorrect responses: Restating the sentence without inferring additional meaning or application. Do you want food? Someone is asking if they're hungry. Have you eaten? Did you have to repeat the bold sentence(s)? Y N If you answered yes, how many times? _____	Correct Meaning? Y N Literal Response? Y N	

CHAPTER 5: ASSESSMENTS FOR THE CONVERSATION FRAMEWORK

Statement	Correct Meaning Or Literal Response? (Y or N)	Hesitation Time in Seconds
9. Is it hot in here to you? What is she really saying? Response: Correct response: Can you turn the air conditioning on/cooler. Turn the heat off, I'm hot. Incorrect responses: Restating the sentence without inferring additional meaning or application. Are you uncomfortable? Are you hot? Did you have to repeat the bold sentence(s)? Y N If you answered yes, how many times? _____	Correct Meaning? Y N Literal Response? Y N	
10. No really … I'm fine. What are they really saying? Response: Correct response: I'm not fine. Incorrect responses: Restating the sentence without inferring additional meaning or application. It's okay. it's not a big deal. Telling someone they're fine. Did you have to repeat the bold sentence(s)? Y N If you answered yes, how many times? _____	Correct Meaning? Y N Literal Response? Y N	

Assessment for Recognizing Idioms and Sarcasm (7 Years – Adult)

Directions: The items on the assessments are read aloud because most conversation is spoken. Read the bold sentence(s) at a regular talking speed. Do not slow down the bold sentence(s) because this may make it easier for the student to identify the topic. Allowable prompts are listed at the top of the assessment.

Read each of the following comments to the student in a monotone voice without much emphasis on the sarcastic content. After reading each item, ask the student to state the correct meaning by asking, "What did she mean?" Once the student has responded, circle Y (Yes) or N (No) in the appropriate column to identify whether the student's response was appropriate for the situation.

Original Comment	Acceptable Response	Appropriate for Situation (Y or N)
Ex: After studying for a long time, Rosa said, "My head is spinning." What did she mean? *Response: "Rosa was so tired that she needed to stop studying."* *Did you have to repeat the bold sentence(s)?* Y (N) *If you answered yes, how many times?* __0__	Acceptable responses: I am very tired; I am so tired that I cannot study any more; I can't think clearly now. Incorrect responses: I don't know; my head is turning around; any literal interpretation.	(Y) N

TALK WITH ME

Original Comment	Acceptable Response	Appropriate for Situation (Y or N)
1. **Leah's mother said, "I really need you to wake up your sister this morning." To wake her up, Leah quickly ran upstairs and banged together pots and pans. Leah's sister got up in a bad mood. Leah's father walked into the room and said, "You shouldn't poke the sleeping bear." What did he mean?** Response: Did you have to repeat the bold sentence(s)? Y N If you answered yes, how many times? _____	Acceptable responses: Don't do something that will provoke a negative response or a fight. Incorrect responses: I don't know; bears are dangerous; If you poke the bear, you'll die; any literal interpretation.	Y N
2. **Bennett is interested in getting a job. He sits every day on the sofa thinking about what type of job he wants. He may want to work at a restaurant or local sports store. He can't make up his mind, so he continues to sit on the sofa. Some would say that he's a real "go-getter." What do they mean?** Response: Did you have to repeat the bold sentence(s)? Y N If you answered yes, how many times? _____	Acceptable responses: He's lazy and doesn't do anything; he was being sarcastic because he is not a "go-getter." Incorrect responses: He can't make up his mind; he goes for what he wants; I don't know; he goes fast.	Y N
3. **Claudia was really frustrated and felt like teachers were bossing her around. She was telling her friend about it and commented, "I mean, do they want to wipe my bottom, too?" What did she mean?** Response: Did you have to repeat the bold sentence(s)? Y N If you answered yes, how many times? _____	Acceptable responses: Teachers are telling her how to do every move, treating her like a baby; They want to do everything for her. Incorrect responses: They want to wipe her bottom; They want to make her work harder; I don't know.	Y N

CHAPTER 5: ASSESSMENTS FOR THE CONVERSATION FRAMEWORK

Original Comment	Acceptable Response	Appropriate for Situation (Y or N)
4. Tyler is the most talkative second grader I've seen. He usually has to move his color behavior card because he's generally talking to Liam, a classmate, and not doing what he's supposed to be doing when the teacher is talking. The other day, Joseph said that Tyler was a "man of few words." What did he mean? Response: Did you have to repeat the bold sentence(s)? Y N If you answered yes, how many times? _____	Acceptable responses: Tyler was a person that likes to talk; Tyler talks too much; Joseph was being sarcastic. Incorrect responses: He doesn't talk much; I don't know; said a couple of short words.	Y N
5. Rob loves golfing. He golfs with his friends every weekend at a country club near his house. Last month, Rob drove by a country club on the other side of town that he liked and decided to start golfing there. He frequently complains to his friend, Steven, about how long the drive is. Steven said, "The grass isn't always greener on the other side." What did he mean? Response: Did you have to repeat the bold sentence(s)? Y N If you answered yes, how many times? _____	Acceptable response: New golf place isn't better; He should have stayed at the one close to home; he doesn't like the new place; he isn't able to play with his friends now. Incorrect response: I don't know; The field might not be as nice; The field is nicer.	Y N
6. Corey was unloading groceries from the car. Two of his roommates arrived home and walked past him and into the house. As the door started to close, Corey said, "Thanks for the help!" What did he mean? Response: Did you have to repeat the bold sentence(s)? Y N If you answered yes, how many times? _____	Acceptable response: Corey was being sarcastic; They weren't helping. Incorrect responses: I don't know; He was thankful; He was thanking them for helping; They helped him; He needed help.	Y N

TALK WITH ME

Original Comment	Acceptable Response	Appropriate for Situation (Y or N)
7. **Ted is a talkative person who has many friends and goes out a lot. John is shy, has few friends, and does not go out often.** One day, John and Ted were fishing in a lake. They left their dock at 5:30 AM and anchored the boat close to the shore. Ted complained to John about having to go to so many activities with everyone he knows. John said, "We're in the same boat." What did John mean? Response: Did you have to repeat the bold sentence(s)? Y N If you answered yes, how many times? _____	Acceptable response: John was being sarcastic because they aren't in the same boat. Incorrect responses: I don't know.	Y N
8. **Tim works at a grocery store.** One day, Tim was talking to Jeff, and a customer knocked over a stack of cereal boxes. When he heard this, Tim ran to go clean up the cereal boxes. Jeff said, "He's really dragging his feet on that one." What did Jeff mean? Response: Did you have to repeat the bold sentence(s)? Y N If you answered yes, how many times? _____	Acceptable response: Jeff was being sarcastic; Tim ran to pick up the cereal boxes; Time was in a hurry; he left the conversation quickly; he wasn't dragging his feet at all. Incorrect responses: I don't know; Tim walked slowly; Tim was shuffling.	Y N
9. **What does sarcasm mean?** Response: Did you have to repeat the bold sentence(s)? Y N If you answered yes, how many times? _____	Acceptable responses: Saying the opposite of what is really meant intended to entertain or insult someone; the use of irony to mock, ridicule, or taunt someone in a joking or hurtful way. Incorrect responses: I don't know; someone joking or being mean with no reference to the other part of the definition; telling a lie.	Y N

CHAPTER 5: ASSESSMENTS FOR THE CONVERSATION FRAMEWORK

BALANCING THE CONVERSATION

Assessment for Balancing Questions, Stories, and Comments

Tally Mark Chart (Two People)

The following assessments measure not only individual ability – a student's ability to balance questions, stories, and comments within 0-2 seconds – but also the abilities of multiple people at once. A consistent lack in one of these three areas indicates a deficit in the student's ability to do the specific task (e.g., ask questions, tell stories, or make comments). Conversational deficits can manifest in many different ways, but they will show up on this chart if the chart is being used correctly and each contribution to the conversation is receiving a tally mark. For students who interrupt frequently, writing an "I" by their name helps track interruptions, which is typically someone entering the conversation at the wrong time.

Directions: Write the names or initials of each student by the numbers to identify each person's individual performance. As the conversation begins, immediately begin tracking the conversation by making a tally mark to track each question, story, and comment.

Student's Name	Questions	Stories	Comments
1.			
2.			

Additional Tally Mark Charts may be found in Appendix Y, with options to complete data collection for 3-8 people participating in the conversation.

ASKING QUESTIONS

This part of the assessment includes detailed information related to a student's ability to ask the three types of questions: (a) questions to start a conversation, (b) follow-up questions, and (c) reciprocal questions.

Questions to Start a Conversation

A large proportion of conversation with someone new consists of asking questions. Asking questions to start a conversation allows you to get to know someone. Proficiency is based on the ability to identify categories of conversation topics quickly and to state those categories within a question.

TALK WITH ME

Assessing skills in this area begins with having the student verbally identify as many topics as he can think of to start a conversation. This skill relies on rote memorization, often an area of strength for individuals with ASD. Again, hesitation time is important.

Assessment for Starting a Conversation With School-Age People You Do Not Know

Directions: Say, "When you meet a person your age, it's important to ask questions. What are three different questions you can ask someone your age whom you've never met?" Acceptable prompts include "You could ask that, but it's probably not the first thing that someone would ask. What is something obvious that you could ask?" Use the Order column to check which topics were introduced first, second, third, and so forth, then jot down the sample question generated by the student as well as the total time.

Topics for Starting a Conversation With School-Age People You Do Not Know Total Time:_____		Sample Question Generated by Student
Order	**Appropriate Topics**	
	Where You Are (right now)	
	Who You Are With (right now)	
	Name	
	Grade/School	
	Hobbies/Interests	
	Other:	
	Other:	
	Other:	

CHAPTER 5: ASSESSMENTS FOR THE CONVERSATION FRAMEWORK

Assessment for Starting a Conversation With Adults You Do Not Know

Directions: Say, "When you meet a new adult, it's important to ask questions. What are three different questions you can ask an adult whom you do not know?" Acceptable prompts include "You could ask that, but it's probably not the first thing that someone would ask. What is something that you could ask a new person?" Use the Order column to check which topics were introduced first, second, third, and so forth, then jot down the sample question generated by the student as well as the total time.

Topics for Starting a Conversation With Adults You Do Not Know Total Time:_____		Sample Question Generated by Student
Order	**Appropriate Topics**	
	Where You Are (right now)	
	Who You Are With (right now)	
	Name	
	Job	
	Hobbies/Interests	
	Other:	
	Other:	
	Other:	

Assessment for Starting a Conversation With People You Know

Directions: Say, "When you're talking with an adult you know, it's important to ask questions. What are three different questions you can ask an adult you know?" Acceptable prompts include "You could ask that, but it's probably not the first thing that someone would ask. What is something that you could ask a new person?" Use the Order column to check which topics were introduced first, second, third, and so forth, then jot down the sample question generated by the student as well as the total time.

TALK WITH ME

Topics for Starting a Conversation With People You Know Total Time:_____		Sample Question Generated by Student
Order	**Appropriate Topics**	
	People/Lives	
	School	
	Job	
	Hobbies/Interests	
	Current Events	
	News	
	Weekend	
	TV Shows	
	Movies	
	Music	
	Electronics	
	Books	
	Places	
	Sports	
	Food	
	Weather	
	Holidays	
	Vacations	
	Family/Pets	
	Where You Are (right now)	
	Who You're With (right now)	
	Weird Things	
	Other:	
	Other:	
	Other:	
	Other:	
	Other:	
	Other:	

CHAPTER 5: ASSESSMENTS FOR THE CONVERSATION FRAMEWORK

Follow-Up Questions

The ability to ask follow-up questions about what someone just said contributes to maintaining a longer conversation. First assess the student's ability to ask follow-up questions when prompted, then unprompted. Topics were selected so that this assessment tool can be used for any age group.

Assessment for Follow-Up Questions – Prompted

Directions: Tell the student that you will be assessing her ability to ask follow-up questions. Explain that a follow-up question is a question about what someone just said. Let her know you will be reading 15 items and that it is her job is to ask three follow-up questions about what you just said. Say, "I'll say a comment, and I want you to ask me three follow-up questions about what I just said." Record the exact responses and hesitation time. Acceptable prompts include "What could you ask me?," "Follow-up question (with gesture prompt to self)," and "What's another follow-up question?" If the student does not ask a follow-up question within 20 seconds, record the hesitation time as "20+" and move on. As appropriate, write the response in the space provided on the form below.

If the student makes a comment, redirect him by saying, "Remember, ask me a question about what *I* just said." Track the hesitation time for each follow-up question and note it in the right-hand column below. The time will start over after the student completes asking a follow-up question and is ready to move on to the next follow-up question.

Random Comments	Student Response/Follow-Up Question	Hesitation Time (sec.)
Ex: "I just finished reading a good book."	1. "What book did you read?" 2. What kind of book is it? 3. What was it about? Off-Topic Comments: _____III_____	1. 14 sec 2. 7 sec 3. 5 sec
1. I can't wait to go to the beach.	1. 2. 3. Off-Topic Comments: _____	1. 2. 3.
2. I just got back from Atlanta.	1. 2. 3. Off-Topic Comments: _____	1. 2. 3.
3. My tooth hurts.	1. 2. 3. Off-Topic Comments: _____	1. 2. 3.

TALK WITH ME

Random Comments	Student Response/Follow-Up Question	Hesitation Time (sec.)
4. My birthday was yesterday.	1. 2. 3. Off-Topic Comments: _____	1. 2. 3.
5. What a long day.	1. 2. 3. Off-Topic Comments: _____	1. 2. 3.
6. I wonder what time the store will close.	1. 2. 3. Off-Topic Comments: _____	1. 2. 3.
7. I hate homework.	1. 2. 3. Off-Topic Comments: _____	1. 2. 3.
8. I need to get a hat.	1. 2. 3. Off-Topic Comments: _____	1. 2. 3.
9. My dad and I went to the Barber Speedway.	1. 2. 3. Off-Topic Comments: _____	1. 2. 3.
10. I hope my dog starts feeling better.	1. 2. 3. Off-Topic Comments: _____	1. 2. 3.
11. I had to go to the hospital yesterday.	1. 2. 3. Off-Topic Comments: _____	1. 2. 3.

CHAPTER 5: ASSESSMENTS FOR THE CONVERSATION FRAMEWORK

Random Comments	Student Response/Follow-Up Question	Hesitation Time (sec.)
12. Hold picture frame with picture in it. (Don't say anything.)	1. 2. 3. Off-Topic Comments: _____	1. 2. 3.
13. I thought I had seen everything until this morning.	1. 2. 3. Off-Topic Comments: _____	1. 2. 3.
14. I am so excited that I can hardly concentrate.	1. 2. 3. Off-Topic Comments: _____	1. 2. 3.
15. I thought I saw a turtle in the middle of the road on my way here.	1. 2. 3. Off-Topic Comments: _____	1. 2. 3.

TALK WITH ME

Assessment for Follow-Up Questions – Unprompted

Directions: If the student did well on the Assessment for Follow-Up Questions – Prompted, move on to this section. When under pressure, some students struggle to ask questions. It is important to be able to ask questions under pressure. You can still complete this even if the student did not do well with the follow-up questions with prompts; however, do not tell the student that you will be assessing his ability to ask follow-up questions. Instead, integrate the comments into your interaction in a natural conversation and record the student's hesitation time. If the students does not ask a follow-up question within 20 seconds, record it as "20+" and move on. As appropriate, write the response in the space provided on the form below. Track the hesitation time for each follow-up question and note it in the right-hand column. The time will start over after the student completes asking a follow-up question and is ready to move on to the next follow-up question.

Random Comments	Student Response/Follow-Up Question	Hesitation Time (sec.)
Ex: Say, " I just finished reading a good book."	Ex: 1. "What book did you read?" 2. "Do you read a lot?" 3. "Have you read the book ___?"	Ex: 1. 8 sec. 2. 15 sec. 3. 7 sec.
1. I can't wait to go to the beach.	1. 2.	1. 2.
2. Our family just got a new dog.	1. 2.	1. 2.
3. My favorite TV show comes on tonight.	1. 2.	1. 2.
4. My birthday is in two days.	1. 2.	1. 2.
5. Today has been the best day!	1. 2.	1. 2.

Reciprocal Questions

Directions: Reciprocal questions are used frequently in small talk and occasionally in longer conversations. It is important to ask reciprocal questions to let others know that you care about them. Say, "I will be asking you some questions, and I want you to ask me a question back." Then, read the original question. Note if an acceptable reciprocal question is asked by circling Y or N and write down the hesitation time in the respective columns. The hesitation time starts the instant the student has finished answering your question. For example, if you ask "Who was your favorite character?," the student would answer your question by telling you his favorite character. As soon as he has given that information, start tracking his hesitation time and note it in the right-hand column. The goal is for each student to answer the question and then ask you a reciprocal question with as little hesitation time as possible.

CHAPTER 5: ASSESSMENTS FOR THE CONVERSATION FRAMEWORK

Assessment for Reciprocal Questions – Prompted

Original Question	Student Response/Reciprocal Question	Hesitation Time (sec.)
Ex: "What is your favorite color?"	Ex: What is your favorite color?; What about you?; You?	Ex: 1 sec
1. How are you?	Acceptable responses: How are you?; What about you?; You? Y N	
2. What are you doing this weekend/What did you do last weekend?	Acceptable responses: What are you doing this weekend?; What about you?; You? Y N	
3. Who is your favorite character in a movie or TV show?	Acceptable responses: Who is yours?; What about you?; You? Y N	
4. What do you like to do?	Acceptable responses: What do you like to do?; What are you into?; What about you? You? Y N	
5. What do you like to do with your friends?	Acceptable responses: What do you like to do with your friends?; What about you?; You? Y N	

Assessment for Reciprocal Questions – Unprompted

Directions: Start a conversation with the student. Ask each of the questions during the conversation. Note if an acceptable reciprocal question is asked by circling Y or N and write down the hesitation time in the respective columns. The hesitation time starts the instant the student has finished answering your question. For example, if you ask, "Who was your favorite character?" the student would answer your question by telling you his favorite character. As soon as he has given that information, start tracking his hesitation time. The goal is for each student to answer the question and then ask you a reciprocal question with as little hesitation time as possible. No prompts should be given.

Original Question	Student Response/Reciprocal Question	Hesitation Time (sec.)
Ex: "Who was your favorite character?"	Ex: "I don't have one. Who was yours?"	Ex: 1 sec
1. How are you?	Acceptable responses: How are you?; What about you?; You? Y N	
2. What did you do today?	Acceptable responses: What did you do today?; What about you?; You? Y N	
3. Have you seen any recent movies?	Acceptable responses: Have you seen any recent movies?; What about you?; You? Y N	
4. How was your day today?	Acceptable responses: How was your day?; What about you?; You? Y N	
5. What are you doing this weekend/ What did you do last weekend?	Acceptable responses: What are you doing this weekend?; What about you? You? Y N	

TELLING STORIES

This part of the assessment includes detailed information related to a student's ability to tell four types of stories: (a) sequential stories, (b) information stories, and (c) emotional stories, and (d) related stories.

Assessment for Sequential Stories

Directions: Choose at least three of the five story prompts. It is important to use story prompts with familiar content to the student (e.g., the example of the snowman may be inappropriate for someone living in a warm climate).. Listen to the student's sequential story and answer the assessment questions by circling Y (Yes) and N (No) for each of the questions, including (a) Did the story have sequential order?, (b) Did the story include relevant details?, (c) Did the story include transitions (first/next, beginning/end)?, and (d) How many sentences were included in the story?

Depending on the student's needs, the Conversation Topics List may or may not be used as a visual support. Note on the assessment when the Conversation Topics List (see Appendix C or D) is used as a visual support. Using this visual support makes identifying the topic easier, but it is important to gradually remove it to ensure that the student can engage in a conversation withouy the visual support available. If the student is working on identifying the topic with background noise, intentional background noise should be used. Circle Y (Yes) or N (No) in the appropriate row at the bottom of the assessment, depending on whether or not intentional background noise was used.

CHAPTER 5: ASSESSMENTS FOR THE CONVERSATION FRAMEWORK

Allowable Prompts: *"Tell me a story." "Can you tell me more?"*		
Story Prompt	**Expectation**	**Rating**
Ex: *"Tell me about your day today."*	Did the story have sequential order?	**Y** N
	Did the story include relevant details?	Y **N**
	Did the story include transitions (first/next, beginning/end)?	Y **N**
	How many sentences were included in the story?	3
NOTES		
1. Tell me what you did this past weekend.	Did the story have a sequential order?	Y N
	Did the story include relevant details?	Y N
	Did the story include transitions (first/next, beginning/end)?	Y N
	How many sentences were included in the story?	
NOTES		
2. Tell me about the last movie or TV show you saw.	Did the story have a sequential order?	Y N
	Did the story include relevant details?	Y N
	Did the story include transitions (first/next, beginning/end)?	Y N
	How many sentences were included in the story?	
NOTES		
3. Tell me how to make a snowman.	Did the story have a sequential order?	Y N
	Did the story include relevant details?	Y N
	Did the story include transitions (first/next, beginning/end)?	Y N
	How many sentences were included in the story?	
NOTES		

Story Prompt	Expectation	Rating
4. Tell me what you did to get ready for school this morning.	Did the story have a sequential order?	Y N
	Did the story include relevant details?	Y N
	Did the story include transitions (first/next, beginning/end)?	Y N
	How many sentences were included in the story?	_____
NOTES		
5. Tell me about a time when you had fun with friends or family.	Did the story have a sequential order?	Y N
	Did the story include relevant details?	Y N
	Did the story include transitions (first/next, beginning/end)?	Y N
	How many sentences were included in the story?	_____
NOTES		
During the assessment, did the student use the Conversation Topics List as a visual support?		Y N
During the assessment, was there intentional background noise?		Y N

Assessment for Informational Stories

Directions: Choose at least three of the five story prompts. It is important to use story prompts with content that is familiar to the student. Listen to the student's informational story and answer the assessment questions by circling Y (Yes) and N (No) for each of the three questions, including (a) Did the story make sense? (b) Did the story include relevant details? and (c) How many sentences were included in the story?

Depending on the student's needs, the Conversation Topics List may or may not be used as a visual support. Note on the assessment when the Conversation Topics List is used as a visual support. Using this visual support makes identifying the topic easier, but it is important to gradually remove it to ensure that the student can engage in a conversation without the visual support available. If the student is working on identifying the topic with background noise, intentional background noise should be used. Circle Y (Yes) or N (No) in the appropriate row at the bottom of the assessment depending on whether or not intentional background noise was used.

CHAPTER 5: ASSESSMENTS FOR THE CONVERSATION FRAMEWORK

Allowable Prompts: *"Tell me a story." "Can you tell me more?" "Can you tell me a story."*		
Story Prompt	**Expectation**	**Rating**
Prompt Ex: *"Tell me about a TV show you like."*	Did the story make sense?	Y (N)
	Did the story include relevant details?	Y (N)
	How many sentences were included in the story?	0
NOTES *Kickin It.*		
1. Tell me how to play a game you like.	Did the story make sense?	Y N
	Did the story include relevant details?	Y N
	How many sentences were included in the story?	___
NOTES		
2. Tell me about a restaurant you like.	Did the story make sense?	Y N
	Did the story include relevant details?	Y N
	How many sentences were included in the story?	___
NOTES		
3. Tell me about your family.	Did the story make sense?	Y N
	Did the story include relevant details?	Y N
	How many sentences were included in the story?	___
NOTES		
4. Tell me what you do in your classroom.	Did the story make sense?	Y N
	Did the story include relevant details?	Y N
	How many sentences were included in the story?	___
NOTES		

Story Prompt	Expectation	Rating
5. Do you have a pet? Tell me about him/her.	Did the story make sense?	Y N
	Did the story include relevant details?	Y N
	How many sentences were included in the story?	_____
NOTES		
During the assessment, did the student use the Conversation Topics List as a visual support?		Y N
During the assessment, was there intentional background noise?		Y N

Assessment for Emotional Stories

Directions: Choose at least three of the five story prompts. It is important to use story prompts with familiar content to the student. Listen to the student's emotional story and answer the assessment questions by circling Y (Yes) and N (No) for each of the three questions, including (a) Did the story make sense? (b) Did the story include relevant details? and (c) How many sentences were included in the story?

Depending on the student's needs, the Conversation Topics List may or may not be used as a visual support. Note on the assessment when the Conversation Topics List is used as a visual support. Using this visual support makes identifying the topic easier, but it is important to gradually remove it to ensure that the student can engage in a conversation without the visual support available. If the student is working on identifying the topic with background noise, intentional background noise should be used. Circle Y (Yes) or N (No) in the appropriate row at the bottom of the assessment, depending on whether or not intentional background noise was used.

Story Prompt	Expectation	Rating
Ex: "Tell me about a time when you were confused."	Did the story make sense?	Y **N**
	Did the story include relevant details?	Y **N**
	How many sentences were included in the story?	0
NOTES		
1. Tell me something that made you feel angry.	Did the story make sense?	Y N
	Did the story include relevant details?	Y N
	How many sentences were included in the story?	_____
NOTES		

CHAPTER 5: ASSESSMENTS FOR THE CONVERSATION FRAMEWORK

Story Prompt	Expectation	Rating
2. Have you ever had something exciting happen to you? Tell me a time that you felt excited.	Did the story make sense?	Y N
	Did the story include relevant details?	Y N
	How many sentences were included in the story?	_____
NOTES		
3. Tell me about a time when you lost something (story should include context associated with disappointed or worried).	Did the story make sense?	Y N
	Did the story include relevant details?	Y N
	How many sentences were included in the story?	_____
NOTES		
4. Tell me about a time when you were very sad.	Did the story make sense?	Y N
	Did the story include relevant details?	Y N
	How many sentences were included in the story?	_____
NOTES		
5. Tell me about the last time you remember being afraid.	Did the story make sense?	Y N
	Did the story include relevant details?	Y N
	How many sentences were included in the story?	_____
NOTES		
During the assessment, did the student use the Conversation Topics List as a visual support?	Y N	
During the assessment, was there intentional background noise?	Y N	

Assessment for Related Stories

Directions: Choose at least three of the five story prompts. It is important to use story prompts with content that is familiar to the student. Listen to the student's related story and answer the assessment questions by circling Y (Yes) and N (No) for each of the three questions, including (a) Did the story make sense? (b) Did the story include relevant details? (c) Was the story on the same topic as the story prompt, and (d) How many sentences were included in the story?

Depending on the student's needs, the Conversation Topics List may or may not be used as a visual support. Note on the assessment when the Conversation Topics List is used as a visual support. Using this visual support makes identifying the topic easier, but it is important to gradually remove it to ensure that the student can engage in a conversation without the visual support available. If the student is working on identifying the topic with background noise, intentional background noise should be used. Circle Y (Yes) or N (No) in the appropriate row at the bottom of the assessment, depending on whether or not intentional background noise was used.

TALK WITH ME

Allowable Prompts: *"Can you tell me a related story?" "Tell me a story." "Can you tell me more?" "The story should be on a similar topic as my story." "What was my story about?" "Tell a story about that."*

Story Prompt	Expectation	Rating
Ex: "Yesterday was really busy for me. After work, I drove an hour to meet someone to buy furniture. Then I drove 30 minutes to meet up with some friends for a birthday dinner. Then I finally got home at 9:00 to do laundry and clean my house because I am having people over tomorrow."	Did the story make sense?	Y (N)
	Did the story include relevant details?	Y (N)
	Was the story on the same topic as the story prompt?	Y (N)
	How many sentences were included in the story?	1

NOTES
I am worried about a real Ice Age and bringing back prehistoric animals. I wonder if we'll have to evolve to get more hair or something.

Story Prompt	Expectation	Rating
1. This weekend I got to hang out with my siblings. There is this new place near my house that has some really great pizza. After eating, we went to a movie and then over to my brother's house. The next day, we all went to church together. Tell a related story.	Did the story make sense?	Y N
	Did the story include relevant details?	Y N
	Was the story on the same topic as the story prompt?	Y N
Related story should be on the topic of: weekend, family, food, or movies	How many sentences were included in the story?	_____

NOTES

Story Prompt	Expectation	Rating
2. Last summer, my parents came to town with an RV. They rented a place at a campground and let my kids spend the night camping. My kids loved it. My parents took tons of pictures of the kids going camping. Tell a related story.	Did the story make sense?	Y N
	Did the story include relevant details?	Y N
	Was the story on the same topic as the story prompt?	Y N
Related story should be on the topic of: family, hobbies/interests, camping, or summer	How many sentences were included in the story?	_____

NOTES

Story Prompt	Expectation	Rating
3. I watched a really strange movie the other day. I'm not completely sure what it was about. It was really slow to start, and I couldn't figure out what the plot was. It was about a kid who had a lot of problems with his family and his friends, but nothing was ever resolved. Tell a related story.	Did the story make sense?	Y N
	Did the story include relevant details?	Y N
	Was the story on the same topic as the story prompt?	Y N
Related story should be on the topic of: movies, family, or weird things	How many sentences were included in the story?	_____

NOTES

CHAPTER 5: ASSESSMENTS FOR THE CONVERSATION FRAMEWORK

Story Prompt	Expectation	Rating
4. I went out to dinner yesterday, and the strangest thing happened. While sitting at the restaurant, I looked over and noticed this person pouring everyone's drinks into his cup. At first I thought it was an employee trying to save trips, but then he drank it. It was so disgusting. Tell a related story. Related story should be on the topic of: people/lives, places, weird things, or disgusting	Did the story make sense?	Y N
	Did the story include relevant details?	Y N
	Was the story on the same topic as the story prompt?	Y N
	How many sentences were included in the story?	_____
NOTES		
5. One time I was in New York on a business trip, and I went to a haunted house. I had seen on TV that it was the scariest haunted house in the United States. It was really neat. I went by myself, but I really wish I went with some people because it was really scary. Tell a related story. Related story should be on the topic of: vacations, places, holidays, Halloween, haunted houses, weird things, scary/scared	Did the story make sense?	Y N
	Did the story include relevant details?	Y N
	Was the story on the same topic as the story prompt?	Y N
	How many sentences were included in the story?	_____
NOTES		
During the assessment, did the student use the Conversation Topics List as a visual support?		Y N
During the assessment, was there intentional background noise?		Y N

MAKING COMMENTS

This final part of the assessment of Balancing Asking Questions, Telling Stories, and Making Comments includes detailed information related to a student's ability to make two types of comments: (a) empathetic comments and (b) response comments.

A student may become successful at conversation without utilizing reflex comments or satirical comments. For that reason, it is not essential to assess these types of comments because they are not required to be proficient in conversation.

Assessment for Empathetic Comments

Directions: Read the original comment to the student. Record the student's response, as well as whether it was a question (Q), story (S), or comment (C). Because this assessment is measuring empathetic comments, note whether the student's comment was appropriate by circling Y (Yes) or N (No). In the last column, record the hesitation time. If the student responds with an on-topic question, say, "Can you make a comment?" If she tells a story or references an off-topic subject, do not provide a prompt. If she is unable to provide a comment, consider the response incorrect by circling N (No).

TALK WITH ME

Original Comment	Response	Hesitation Time (sec.)
Ex: Everyone got their work into the art exhibit except for me. I worked hard on that assignment. **Acceptable response:** Any reference to: I'm sorry; Sounds disappointing; That must be frustrating.	Comment: *You must be so disappointed.* | Q | S | C | Y N	Ex: 2 sec *1 sec*
1. We put my dog to sleep yesterday. **Acceptable response:** Any reference to: I'm sorry; I'm sorry to hear that; That's awful; Which one? Oh no!	Comment: | Q | S | C | Y N	
2. My uncle just got diagnosed with cancer. **Acceptable response:** Any reference to: I'm so sorry to hear that; I'll be praying for him; That's a shock.	Comment: | Q | S | C | Y N	

Original Comment	Response	Hesitation Time (sec.)
3. I wasn't able to study for the test. **Acceptable response:** Any reference to: That's no good; That stinks.	Comment: | Q | S | C | Y N	
4. I left my lunch at home. (Unless it would be a satirical comment between friends) **Acceptable response:** Any reference to: Hope you can get something; Sorry about that.	Comment: | Q | S | C | Y N	
5. I can't wait for volleyball tryouts. I hope I make the team. **Acceptable response:** Any reference to: Good luck; I hope you make it; You'll do well.	Comment: | Q | S | C | Y N	

CHAPTER 5: ASSESSMENTS FOR THE CONVERSATION FRAMEWORK

Assessment for Response Comments

Directions: Read the comment to the student and record the response, as well as whether it was a question (Q), story (S), or comment (C). Then note whether the comment was appropriate by circling Y (Yes) or N (No) and record the hesitation time.

If the student responds with an on-topic question, say, "Can you make a comment?" If she tells a story or references an off-topic subject, do not provide a prompt. If she is unable to provide a comment, consider the response incorrect and circle N.

Original Comment	Response			Hesitation Time (sec.)
Ex: I don't remember the password and I need to check my email. **Acceptable Comments** Any reference to: That's no good, hate that, hope you'll remember it.	Comment: *Oh, that's a pain.* | Q | S | C | | | | I | (Y) N			Ex: 2 sec 3 sec

Original Comment	Response			Hesitation Time (sec.)
1. My cousins are coming in town today.= **Acceptable Comments** Any reference to: Cool, sounds fun, have fun.	Comment: | Q | S | C | | | | | Y N			
2. My back hurts. **Acceptable Comments** Any reference to: So am I, Sorry, that's not good, hope it gets better.	Comment: | Q | S | C | | | | | Y N			
3. I can't wait for my birthday to get here. **Acceptable Comments** Any reference to: That's exciting, sounds like fun.	Comment: | Q | S | C | | | | | Y N			
4. I am going to get my teaching re-certification today. **Acceptable Comments** Any reference to: That's awesome, good luck.	Comment: | Q | S | C | | | | | Y N			

Original Comment	Response	Hesitation Time (sec.)
5. I couldn't find what I wanted at the store yesterday. **Acceptable Comments** Any reference to: That's no good, that's no fun, hate that, hope you'll find it.	Comment: | Q | S | C | |---|---|---| | | | | Y N	
6. I'm looking forward to the weekend. **Acceptable Comments** Any reference to: Me too, cool!	Comment: | Q | S | C | |---|---|---| | | | | Y N	
7. My dog ran away before school this morning. I found him by the garage door when I was pulling out of my driveway. **Acceptable Comments** Any reference to: That's annoying, glad he's back home.	Comment: | Q | S | C | |---|---|---| | | | | Y N	
8. I couldn't find anyone to go skating. **Acceptable Comments** Any reference to: That stinks, maybe you'll be able to find someone, hope you can find something else to do.	Comment: | Q | S | C | |---|---|---| | | | | Y N	
9. I went to the movies last weekend, but they were sold out. **Acceptable Comments** Any reference to: That stinks.	Comment: | Q | S | C | |---|---|---| | | | | Y N	
10. My son got his braces off last week. **Acceptable Comments** Any reference to: Awesome, that's cool, I bet he's happy.	Comment: | Q | S | C | |---|---|---| | | | | Y N	

CHAPTER 5: ASSESSMENTS FOR THE CONVERSATION FRAMEWORK

BRIDGING THE TOPIC

Assessment for Bridging the Topic

Directions: Choose three of the five starting topics for assessment. It is important to use starting topics with familiar content to the student. Say, "We are going to do an activity to see how well you do with changing topics. I will give you the starting topic. You need to tell me at least three different ways you would use 'Speaking of …' to gradually change the subject to another topic without it being a huge topic change. For example, if we were talking about math, you'd need to tell me how you could change the topic from math to a related topic." Mark the student's response by entering the topic under Topics in the first column and then circling Y (Yes) or N (No) in response to the questions. If the student is able to give details only about the topic itself, he is maintaining the topic rather than bridging the topic, so this would be incorrect.

Starting Topic	Expectation	Rating
Example: Swimming in a cold pool *Examples:* Speaking of weird things, … Speaking of the weather, … Speaking of hobbies, … Speaking of sports, … Speaking of other things to do, … *Topics:* 1. Speaking of swimming, I went swimming (still on the same topic of swimming) 2. Speaking of swimming, I like diving boards (still on the same topic of pool) 3. Speaking of a pool, I have swum in a hotel pool (still on the same topic of swimming/pool)	Did the student name at least three related topics?	Y **(N)**
	Did the student use transition wording (e.g., speaking of …, that reminds me of …)?	Y **(N)**
	Did the student make a smooth transition?	Y **(N)**
1. Minecraft (other video games, hobbies/interests, weekend) Topics: 1. _____ 2. _____ 3. _____	Did the student name at least three related topics?	Y N
	Did the student use transition wording (e.g., speaking of …, that reminds me of …)?	Y N
	Did the student make a smooth transition?	Y N
2. Church Examples: Speaking of things to do with family, … Speaking of the weekend, … Speaking of other things to do, … Topics: 1. _____ 2. _____ 3. _____	Did the student name at least three related topics?	Y N
	Did the student use transition wording (e.g., speaking of …, that reminds me of …)?	Y N
	Did the student make a smooth transition?	Y N

TALK WITH ME

Starting Topic	Expectation	Rating
3. Beach Examples: Speaking of family, … Speaking of vacations, … Speaking of hobbies, … Speaking of holidays (e.g. summer), … Speaking of other things to do, … Topics: 1. _____ 2. _____ 3. _____	Did the student name at least three related topics?	Y N
	Did the student use transition wording (e.g., speaking of …, that reminds me of …)?	Y N
	Did the student make a smooth transition?	Y N
4. Football game Examples: Speaking of sports, … Speaking of things going on (people/lives), … Speaking of the news, … Speaking of family, … Speaking of hobbies, … Speaking of other things to do, … Topics: 1. _____ 2. _____ 3. _____	Did the student name at least three related topics?	Y N
	Did student use transition wording (e.g., speaking of …, that reminds me of …)?	Y N
	Did the student make a smooth transition?	Y N
5. *Phineas & Ferb* Examples: Speaking of TV shows, … Speaking of weird things, … Speaking of other things to do (people/lives or hobbies/interests), … Topics: 1. _____ 2. _____ 3. _____	Did the student name at least three related topics?	Y N
	Did student use transition wording (e.g., speaking of …, that reminds me of …)?	Y N
	Did the student make a smooth transition?	Y N

CHAPTER 6
STRATEGIES FOR TEACHING THE CONVERSATION FRAMEWORK

By this point, you are knowledgeable about the three steps of the Conversation Framework and are ready to start implementing them. This chapter will introduce teaching strategies designed to help teachers, other professionals, and parents to implement the Conversation Framework. Use of prompts to guide conversation will also be discussed. Specifically, the following five required tools will be described (a) Conversation Topics List, (b) Fast-Paced Audio Recordings, (c) Tally Mark Chart, (d) Bridge Visual, and (e) Transition Cards.

One of the things that make the Conversation Framework different from other programs is its focus on teaching conversation in a natural setting. That is, conversations are structured as little as possible while allowing the instructor to maintain control of the group well enough for the conversation to still be appropriate. be used within natural conversation and drills.

Table 6.1 provides as overview of the teaching strategies and their relationship to the Conversation Framework.

Table 6.1
Overview of the Teaching Strategies and Their Relationship to the Conversation Framework

		Description	Activities	Visual Supports	Assessments
Step 1		**Identify the Topic** Knowing the topic is the first step toward having an effective conversation. To identify the topic, you must be able to identify the subject of a conversation, the weight or seriousness of what is being discussed, the implied emotion within the conversation, and the inferred meaning of the conversation. The concept of "on topic" vs. "off topic" is also addressed.	• How Many • Main Topic • Fast-Paced Audio Recordings	• Conversation Topics List (Appendices C and D) • Tally Mark Chart (Appendix Y)	• Assessment for Identifying the Topic (4 - 11 Years) • Assessment for Identifying the Topic (12 Years - Adult) • Assessment for Girls Conversation (12 Years - Adult) • Assessment for Implied Emotions (5 Years - 12 Years) • Assessment for Implied Emotions (12 Years - Adult) • Assessment for Inferred Meaning (12 Years - Adult) • Assessment for Recognizing Idioms and Sarcasm (7 Years - Adult)

	Description	**Activities**	**Visual Supports**	**Assessments**
Step 2	**Balance Asking Questions, Telling Stories, and Making Comments Within 0-2 Seconds** The term balance is used here to refer to creating an equal distribution of questions, stories, and comments – both with regard to one's own utterances and in proportion to others' statements. **Balance Asking Questions Within 0-2 Seconds** Asking questions is essential to keeping a conversation going. There are three types of questions: (a) questions to start a conversation, (b) follow-up questions about what someone just said, and (c) reciprocal questions. Asking questions allows you to find out information from others, as well as let someone know you are interested in what they have to say. In general, people like to talk about themselves and their experiences. There are times we may not be interested in what someone has to say, but we ask a question anyway because it shows interest in others. **Balance Telling Stories Within 0-2 Seconds** Telling stories is a significant component of having a conversation. Conversations without stories are boring. Stories can be based on sequential, informational, or emotional events. There are two types of stories: (a) stories to start a conversation and (b) related stories. Stories allow you to give information in a logical format. They vary in length.	• Give 3 • Fast-Paced Audio Recordings • Hot Seat • Question Game • Advanced Question Game • Last One Standing • Related Stories • Story Pop • "That Sounds"	• Conversation Topics List • Tally Mark Chart • Carrier Phrases for Asking Questions (Appendix L) • Carrier Phrases for Telling Stories (Appendix M) • Scripts for Comments (Appendix N) • Questions, Stories, Comments, Cheat Sheet 1 (Appendix O) • Questions, Stories, Comments, Cheat Sheet 2 (Appendix P)	• Tally Mark Chart (Two People) • Tally Mark Chart (Three People) • Tally Mark Chart (Four People) • Tally Mark Chart (Five People) • Tally Mark Chart (Six People) • Tally Mark Chart (Seven People) • Tally Mark Chart (Eight People) • Topics for Starting a Conversation With School-Age People You Do Not Know • Topics for Starting a Conversation With Adults You Do Not Know • Assessment for Questions to Start a Conversation With People You Know • Assessment for Follow-Up Questions – Prompted • Assessment for Follow-Up Questions – Unprompted • Assessment for Reciprocal Questions – Prompted • Assessment for Reciprocal Questions – Unprompted • Assessment for Sequential Story • Assessment for Informational Story • Assessment for Emotional Story • Assessment for Story to Start Conversation • Assessment for Related Story • Assessment for Empathetic Comments • Assessment for Response Comments

CHAPTER 6: STRATEGIES FOR TEACHING THE CONVERSATION FRAMEWORK

	Description	Activities	Visual Supports	Assessments
	Balance Making Comments Within 0-2 Seconds Making relevant comments is an important part of mastering conversation. Making comments allows you to show interest in what others are saying and makes others feel comfortable. There are four types of comments: (a) reflex comments, (b) empathetic comments, (c) response comments, and (d) sarcastic comments.			
Step 3	**Bridge the Topic** Bridging the topic is the most vital skill for maintaining a longer conversation. Once the other areas of the Conversation Framework are mastered, the next step is learning to bridge from one topic to a related topic without appearing to make a drastic change in the conversation. There are three types of bridging topics: (a) expanding categories, (b) condensing categories, and (c) smooth transitions.	• Bridging the Topic	• Conversation Topics List • Bridge Visual (Appendix Q) • Common Categories Chart (Appendix R) • Transition Cards (Appendix S)	• Assessment for Bridging Topics

METHODS FOR TEACHING THE CONVERSATION FRAMEWORK

The framework is taught in steps. Each of the five required tools is introduced in a specific order.

1. Administer and analyze individual assessment to determine what to teach.
2. Before beginning the Conversation Framework, show your student the overview of the Conversation Framework (see Appendix B). This will help him to visualize the entire process.
3. Once your student is familiar with the three steps of the Conversation Framework, explain the Conversation Topics List (see Appendix C or D). This visual support will be used during all steps within the Conversation Framework to help the student to know what he is working on first and what he will be working on next.
4. Practice identifying the topic with the student until mastery. If needed, use fast-paced audio recordings (see pages 124-129) as a supplemental resource for all steps within the Conversation Framework, and especially the step for identifying the topic.

5. Once the student is proficient at identifying the topic, use the Tally Mark Chart (see Appendix T or Y) to help the student see the balance between asking questions, telling stories, and making comments. Do this until the student has achieved mastery.
6. Utilize individual drills (similar to assessments in Chapter 5) if your student needs additional practice with asking questions, telling stories, or making comments within 0-2 seconds. Do this until the student has achieved mastery.
7. Once the student is proficient at balancing the conversation by asking questions, telling stories, and making comments within 0-2 seconds, explain the Bridge Visual or Transition Cards (see Appendices Q and S). These tools will help the student to visualize how to bridge the topic.
8. Practice bridging the topic with the student until mastery. Use the Bridge Visual and Transition Cards (see Appendices Q and S) as a resource for developing this skill.

Tips for Working With Younger Children

When working with younger children, be sure that your strategies are engaging. For example, make sure that you are using vocabulary that a younger child understands. Also, it is important to repeat terms that you will be using. The following is an example of a possible way to teach these terms.

- Everyone say, "Conversation."
  (Wait for them to say, "Conversation." Make sure everyone says it.)

- What is *conversation*?
  (Allow all the students to guess if they want to guess. Specifically ask anyone that is new to the group or is trying to learn this term.)

- Conversation is just talking. It's easy. There's three ways that I'm going to help you to have a conversation.
  Everyone say, "Questions."
  (Wait for them to say, "Questions." Make sure everyone says it.)
  Everyone say, "Stories."
  (Wait for them to say, "Stories." Make sure everyone says it.)
  Everyone say, "Comments."
  (Wait for them to say, "Comments." Make sure everyone says it.)
  Those are the three parts of conversation – questions, stories, and comments.

- Ask someone to tell a story (about what they did today, what they like to do, a video game they like to play, etc.).

- Ask a student who is working on asking questions, "What can you ask him/her?"
  (IF NEEDED) If you didn't hear him, say, "Can you please repeat that?" (You can also use fast-paced audio recordings, with permission, if this student is working on listening to peers.

- Say to another student, "Now you tell a related story. I ..."
  (Continue to structure the conversation. Have every student practice multiple questions, stories, and comments while keeping a normal flow to the conversation.)

Younger students need the conversation to be structured, so they will practice correctly. If they practice incorrectly, it will reinforce incorrect habits.

CHAPTER 6: STRATEGIES FOR TEACHING THE CONVERSATION FRAMEWORK

REQUIRED TOOLS

We will now look at each of the five required tools in more detail.

Conversation Topics List

The Conversation Topics List (see Appendix C or D) is a visual overview of conversation topics to be used during conversations. The list includes 22 general topics and is used to help the student to break down conversation topics into categories. For example, this is helpful when identifying the topic during Step 1, deciding what to talk about during Step 2, or bridging the topic during Step 3.

The goal is for each student to memorize the list. Once the list is memorized, the visual support has become a mental image in the student's mind and the printed Conversation Topics List is no longer needed. The list is *only for the students who need it.* If a student knows the list, this support will not help him. In fact, if having to use it, such a student might feel belittled and less likely to participate.

During Step 1

1. Determine the student's difficulty with seeing the big picture and general conversation topics. This can be done formally or informally. This step is more meaningful if you can use real examples of a time when the student focused on details rather than the big picture. Some students with high-functioning autism spectrum disorder (HF-ASD) are aware of their interest in details rather than the big picture. It is important during this step to get the student to agree that the ability to see the big picture can help. Refer to the section on motivation in Chapter 2 for strategies on how to accomplish this.

2. Teach the concept of a topic. Say, "A topic is the main idea of what someone is talking about." Have the Conversation Topics List available during this step. Connect the term *topic* to the words on the list.

3. Give each student a copy of the Conversation Topics List and ask them to begin to memorize it. Explain the simplicity of the list – only 22 topics to memorize. Emphasize that memorizing the topics will help compensate for times when the student's brain blanks out, when he is not sure what others are talking about, or not sure what to say. For durability, create a laminated copy of the Conversation Topics List for the classroom or home setting. (Heavy-duty lamination works best because students often bend and wrinkle handouts, making them difficult to use.)

4. Tell your student to study the list and that afterwards you will ask him to name at least three things on the list. Give the student a few minutes to try to memorize the list. Then say, "Tell me three topics you can talk about." If the student is not able to name topics from the list, have him repeat a few topics after you say them.

5. Using material (e.g., a natural conversation, assessment from Chapter 5, or fast-paced audio recording), ask, "What is the topic?" Allow the student to refer to the Conversation Topics List.

6. Praise correct responses. Redirect incorrect responses. Typically, a student who is unfamiliar with the Conversation Topics List will give a very specific detail of the conversation rather than a general conversation topic.

7. If the student gives a specific detail within the conversation, prompt by saying, "Which general topic would that fall under?"

8. If the student is unable to label the general topic, go down each item on the topic list one-by-one and ask, "Would that be under the topic of people/lives?" Then say, "Would that be under the topic of school?, " and so on. Once the student gets the hang of it, you can simplify your question to a one-word question such as, "Job?" Request a "yes" or "no" response when you name each topic on the list.

9. If you would like the student to go down the items in the Conversation Topics List independently, have him use a pen or pencil to mark on a paper copy of the list or a dry-erase marker to put a dot by the topics on a laminated copy of the list.

During Step 2

1. Have the Conversation Topics List (see Appendix C or D) available – whether on paper, bulletin board, or wall art. By this step, the list should be memorized. Regardless, have it available somewhere in the room.

2. When a student is first beginning to start a conversation with others, tell the student to pick a topic from the list. The student should begin to talk about a general topic. If she begins to talk about a very specific topic, typically a preferred interest, explain the difference between a specific topic and a general topic and prompt the student to choose a general topic.

3. As each topic is introduced, give the student an opportunity, in an individual or a group setting, to practice asking questions from each topic. Some students need examples and modeling before they are able to generate questions on their own.

4. As each topic is introduced, give the student an opportunity, in an individual or a group setting, to practice telling stories from each topic. Some students need examples and modeling before they are able to tell stories on their own.

5. Continue to have the Conversation Topics List available during natural conversations until it is no longer needed. (Laminated copies of the Conversation Topics List for each group participant may be used to make participation easier.)

During Step 3

1. Have the Conversation Topics List (see Appendix C or D) available. Even if the list was memorized during Step 1 or 2, it is important to have it available for reference during this step because you are introducing a difficult skill.

2. Refer to the Bridge Visual (see Appendix Q) to aid the student in bridging the topic.

3. Have Transition Cards (see Appendix S) available as well. Some students understand the Bridge Visual better, but others understand the Transition Cards better.

4. When a student or a group of students is/are continuing a conversation for too long, have them practice bridging the topic. It is important to practice this every time a topic has gone on for too long because otherwise the students are practicing conversation incorrectly. There is no criterion for "too long." Use your professional judgment to determine when a conversation is becoming too lengthy based on listener interest and attention.

5. Write the topic being discussed or the topic you want to start with at the top of the Bridge Visual. Ask the student(s) what the topic could fall under from the Conversation Topics List. After they have identified all the possible topics, have them bridge the topic to one of the topics using the script of, "Speaking of_____, that reminds me of_____." If this script is not appropriate for your student, use another script that is appropriate – that is, something that would be normal for someone of any age to say in conversation.

Fast-Paced Audio Recordings

Teachers and speech-language pathologists (SLPs) sometimes comment that, "It's hard to replicate a conversation" when working with a student individually or "He does not fit with any peer group at our school." Similarly, parents sometimes comment, "We do not have friends or neighbors who come to the house to practice conversation."

One way to solve this problem is to use fast-paced audio recordings. Many conversations that you hear around you can be recorded. Other options for capturing conversations include (a) recording talk radio programs, if you can find radio hosts who talk about current topics that are age appropriate for your student; (b) getting permission to audio record neurotypical students talking about current topics, or (c) using conversation-based podcasts. Today's technology makes this easy at the touch of a button. Fast-paced audio recordings provide the opportunity for repeated practice because students can listen to the recording as many times as necessary to develop conversation skills.

During Steps 1, 2, and 3

1. Develop a fast-paced recording, using any of the options mentioned above, as long as the topic is age appropriate.

2. To use this tool during an individual session, explain what the student is expected to do when you push "pause;" for example, identify the topic, ask a follow-up question, tell a related story, make a comment, or bridge the topic.

3. Play a portion of the fast-paced audio recording.

4. Once you think the student has heard enough information to be able to carry out what he is expected to, push "pause" on the fast-paced audio recording.

5. Point to the student and start counting seconds in your head. Do not give any verbal prompts. The only allowable prompt is a gesture prompt of pointing to the student, so he is aware that he is to contribute at the moment. As a reminder, the student should already know that you will be pointing to him and what he is expected to do (i.e., identify the topic, ask a follow-up question, tell a related story, make a comment, bridge the topic).

6. Remember that the goal is for the student to perform the expected skill within 0-2 seconds, whether this is identifying the topic, asking a follow-up question, telling a related story, making a comment, or bridging the topic. If the hesitation time is any longer in a natural setting, he will have missed the opportunity to contribute to the conversation. Please refer to Chapter 5 for information on data collection. It is important to keep data on hesitation time. Stop counting as soon as the student provides a response.

7. If the student is not able to contribute within 1 minute, repeat #2. After re-explaining what he is expected to do, replay the same portion of the fast-paced audio recording.

8. If he is still unable to contribute in a timely manner, use the same fast-paced audio recording as a teaching tool to go over in detail how to perform the skill requested (i.e., identify the topic, ask a follow-up question, tell a related story, make a comment, bridge the topic). Then make sure the student understands by using another fast-paced audio recording to practice the skill. If the student is not able to contribute within a minute, start over at #2.

9. If the student becomes frustrated during the process, validate his feelings. Remind him that you are there to help and that he can listen to the recording as many times as needed. Point out that the reason why you do not want to give him the answer is that if you give him the answers, it will be hard for him to figure it out for himself in the future and you know he can learn it. If this does not calm the student, take a break and continue the session at a different time – that might mean after 5 minutes or a week.

TALK WITH ME

Conversation Example With Prompts

The following example shows how prompts are used within an individual session. Throughout our sessions, we use a combination of verbal and visual prompts. The prompts are used to guide, redirect, refocus, and encourage students.

NOTE: *The same audio clip was used for two students in back-to-back individual sessions. The following illustrates the difference in the skills they were working on within their sessions. The first student (Gage) had a hard time identifying the topic.*

Setting: Individual setting with student and teacher

Materials: Voice recording from talk radio on last night's Super Bowl halftime show with Katy Perry

Student 1

Age: 17 years old

Gender: Male

Group Size: 1 student (individual session)

Conversational Goals: Gage – Step 1: Identifying the Topic

Strategy for Teaching the Conversation Framework:

Fast-Paced Audio Recording

Student's Responses	Adult Prompts
NOTE: We listened to a 37-second clip (Katy Perry's halftime show – discussed technology and lip syncing, floating above ground on platform, spectacular)	
	Mrs. Kerry: What's the topic? (After listening to it for the first time.)
Gage: I have no idea.	
NOTE: We listened to the 37-second clip again. Mrs. Kerry: What's the topic? (After listening to it for a second time.)	
Gage: Something about a video game.	
NOTE: We listened to the 37-second clip again. Mrs. Kerry: What's the topic? (After listening to it for a third time.)	
Gage: Singer.	
NOTE: We listened to the 37-second clip again. Mrs. Kerry: What's the topic? (After listening to it for a fourth time.)	
Gage: Entertainment	
NOTE: We listened to the 37 second clip yet again. Mrs. Kerry: What's the topic? (After listening to it for a fifth time.)	
Gage: I didn't get anything new.	
NOTE: We went back and listened to one sentence at a time.	
	Voice recording: It was the most technological Super Bowl ever. Mrs. Kerry: What did they say?

CHAPTER 6: STRATEGIES FOR TEACHING THE CONVERSATION FRAMEWORK

Student's Responses	Adult Prompts
Gage: I'm not 100% sure. I don't know what they're talking about.	
	Mrs. Kerry: Most technological Super Bowl ever …
Gage: I wasn't hearing them say bowl; I heard them say pole, I was like … what? So they are talking about the super bowl.	
	Voice recording: Can't top it over the technology that got used.
Gage: I know they are talking about technology there.	
	Mrs. Kerry: What about it though?
Gage: That it couldn't be topped. I didn't watch it, so I don't really know.	
	Mrs. Kerry: Okay. So, so far, the main topic is what?
Gage: The technology used at the Super Bowl.	
	Mrs. Kerry: Yes! Is it easier when we break it down?
Gage: It's still confusing.	
	Voice recording: I like to hear the person sing. There were times that I couldn't figure out if she was lip syncing or not. Mrs. Kerry: What are they talking about?
Gage: They want to hear lip syncing, and I really don't know. It's kind of hard to know the topic when you're not that interested in it.	
	Mrs. Kerry: So you're telling me that you wouldn't be interested in the halftime show if it looked like a video game?
Gage: I don't know. I didn't see it, so I don't know.	
	Mrs. Kerry: Okay. You will have a lot more opportunities if you are able to know the topic even if you aren't interested.
Gage: It's kind of hard to contribute to that conversation if I didn't watch it.	
	Mrs. Kerry: Why?
Gage: I didn't watch the Super Bowl, so I wouldn't know what to talk about.	
	Mrs. Kerry: Even if you have not watched it, you can still know what to talk about by asking questions. What questions can you ask?
Gage: I really wouldn't have any.	
	Mrs. Kerry: We're going to think of three. First, what can you ask me?

Student's Responses	Adult Prompts
Gage: Yeah, I got nothing.	
	Mrs. Kerry: What can you ask me about the technology and Super Bowl?
Gage: I already know about the technology they used.	
	Mrs. Kerry: But you didn't see it.
Gage: I know the technology that they used, but I haven't seen it.	
	Mrs. Kerry: What's the category of conversation?
Gage: Sports and news in the same thing.	
	Mrs. Kerry: Could be. What else could it be?
Gage: Could be entertainment.	
	Mrs. Kerry: So, what could you say to get a conversation going with me on that topic?
Gage: *(looked confused)*	
	Mrs. Kerry: You could say, "Mrs. Kerry, did you watch the halftime show?" You don't have to know about the halftime show to ask me that. You're asking about me – my life and experiences.
Gage: Why would I ask that if I haven't seen it? Then you'd just start talking about it and I wouldn't have any idea if it was true or not.	
	Mrs. Kerry: Conversation is meant to get information, give information, and to make others feel comfortable. In this situation, if you asked me if I'd seen the Super Bowl halftime show, you'd be working on getting information and making others feel comfortable. So it would be important to ask about me even if you're not able to "give information." Does that make sense?
Gage: Yes, but then it would be an awkward conversation.	
	Mrs. Kerry: Why?
Gage: Because I wouldn't have watched it. I wouldn't be able to. If you can't contribute to the conversation, then why are you in the conversation.	
	Mrs. Kerry: Because conversation is sometimes just to get information from someone. In this situation, you'd be getting information from me. Just because we start by talking about the halftime show doesn't mean that is the only thing we'd have to talk about. I know we haven't started working on it yet, but you'd be able to bridge that topic back out to the general category of sports, news, or entertainment and talk about something that you know more about in one of those categories.

CHAPTER 6: STRATEGIES FOR TEACHING THE CONVERSATION FRAMEWORK

Student's Responses	Adult Prompts
Pause	
	Mrs. Kerry: Nothing?
Gage: Yeah.	
	Mrs. Kerry: It's just the right thing to do. You need to ask me questions about it.
Gage: Ah. I just don't really watch football.	
	Mrs. Kerry: Are we talking about football?
Gage: Well, we are talking about my conversation skills and are talking about the halftime show.	
	Mrs. Kerry: On the conversation categories, this would also fall under "people/lives," so you'd find out about me. What can you ask me on topic?
Gage: Uh. Was it a good game?	
	Mrs. Kerry: Ask me about the halftime show since that is what was being discussed.
Gage: So what did they do during the halftime show?	
	Mrs. Kerry: Perfect!
Gage: Even though I'm not interested in that topic. It just feels awkward.	
	Mrs. Kerry: And it will feel awkward until you get the hang of it. Asking questions about the other person, even when you're not interested, is important.

Student 2

Age: 17 years old

Gender: Male

Group Size: 1 student (individual session)

Conversational Goals: Andrew – Step 1: Identifying the Topic

Strategy for Teaching the Conversation Framework

Fast-Paced Audio Recording

Student's Responses	Adult Prompts
NOTE: We listened to a 37-second clip (Katy Perry's halftime show – discussed technology and lip syncing, floating above ground on platform, spectacular)	
	Mrs. Kerry: What's the topic?
Andrew: It was about Katy Perry's performance at the Super Bowl last night.	
	Mrs. Kerry: Perfect.
Andrew: I watched it before I went to bed. Did you see it?	

Tally Mark Chart

The Tally Mark Chart (see Appendices T and Y) is designed to help students learn to balance the three parts of conversation: asking questions, telling stories, and making comments (Step 2 of the Conversation Framework). This visual support allows a group of students to see the number of times they are adding to a conversation using questions, stories, and comments. This is important because students who do not talk much typically do not realize they are not contributing enough to the conversation. In the same way, a student who talks more than everyone else combined typically does not notice that he talks too much. A lot of times, rigid or "stuck" thinking causes a student with HF-ASD to believe that you are wrong when you say that he talks too much or too little. The Tally Mark Chart eliminates that argument. You can ask a student if he has been talking as much as everyone else, and he can see how much he has been talking. The goal is for the student to balance the conversation with himself as well as with everyone else in the group. Please refer to Chapter 4 for an explanation of balancing the conversation.

NOTE: The Tally Mark Chart is not used during Steps 1 or 3 of the Conversation Framework.

During Step 2

1. Begin with a Tally Mark Chart (see Appendices T and Y), either presented on a piece of paper or a dry-erase board.
2. Draw an example conversation on the paper or dry-erase board to discuss the concept of "balancing" the conversation. Tell the students that they need to balance the conversation with themselves as well as with everyone else. Ask questions to ensure the expectations are understood before you get started. With younger children or children who are unfamiliar with the concept of "balance," spend time drawing examples of tally marks on a see-saw and illustrate how many tally marks it would take to make it balanced and unbalanced. Ask, "Is this balanced?" and allow students to respond.
3. Once the students understand the concept of balance using tally marks, write each student's name down the left-hand side of the chart. The Tally Mark Chart rows should equal the exact number of group participants expected to contribute to the conversation. Determine the order of names that works best for you as you collect tally marks (e.g., write names in order that the students are seated from left to right). Use the same strategy for ordering names each time you use a Tally Mark Chart. This will make it easier for you to efficiently track data.
4. Ask a student to start the conversation. If someone says, "Let's talk about summer," tell them that is too formal and that they just need to start the conversation randomly because that is what people do.
5. Once the students begin talking naturally, write a tally mark in the correct column each time a student contributes to the conversation correctly using a question, story, or comment.

Conversation Example With Prompts

The following example shows how prompts are used within a natural conversation. Throughout our sessions, we use a combination of verbal and visual prompts. The prompts are used to guide, redirect, refocus, and encourage students.

Age: 8 - 9 years old

Gender: Male

Group Size: 3 students

Conversational Goals:
  Will – Step 2: Balancing the Conversation (Including Telling Stories and Making Comments)
  Alex – Step 2: Balancing the Conversation (Including Asking Questions)
  Cody – Step 2: Balancing the Conversation (Including Asking Follow-Up Questions)

Strategy for Teaching the Conversation Framework
  Natural Conversation

CHAPTER 6: STRATEGIES FOR TEACHING THE CONVERSATION FRAMEWORK

Students' Conversation	Adult Prompts
Will: Hey guys, so uh, do you guys have a Nobby? Alex: No, I don't have a Nobby. Cody: Hey, Will, what is a Nobby? Alex: My mom has a Nook though. It's like the ones in the library. Cody: Oh, like a tablet? Alex: Yeah, the ones in the library. Will: It's … it's … I have a Nobby and the games. In the morning I play my Nobby on the bus, and the games I have on there are the first Typermon, Jetpack Joyride, Angry Birds, and Star Wars Angry Birds. I also have Subway Surfers and Survival Craft. Alex: Survival Craft yeah. Will: So guys, hey uh, do you guys have like a Kindle or iPad? Alex: My dad has an iPad, and my mom has a tablet Nook. Cody: I have a tablet, and I got a DS [Nintendo]. I think I'll show it to you. It's charging. Will: My aunt is getting me a Kindle for Christmas. Alex: A Kindle Fire? Will: Yes, a Kindle Fire.	
	Mrs. Kerry: Okay, let's look at how balanced you are this time (pointing at dry-erase board with Tally Mark Chart). See Will, you didn't have to ask questions the whole time. You do have to ask some. This was perfect. You asked some questions and told some stories. This is looking balanced so far.
Will: I'm sorry.	
	Mrs. Kerry: You have nothing to apologize for because this looks perfect. I just wanted to stop you to say to keep doing it like this. This is exactly right. You have 1 – 1 – 1. He has 2 – 2 – 1. He has 0 – 1 – 3. So far, you guys are pretty close. If you had to do one thing, what would it be?
Alex: Um, ask questions.	
	Mrs. Kerry: For Alex specifically so he has something in that box. Yes.
Cody: Compromise.	
	Mrs. Kerry: Compromise, yes. It's a good thing to compromise, but we don't really need to compromise in conversation.

TALK WITH ME

Students' Conversation	Adult Prompts
Cody: But you take turns.	
	Mrs. Kerry: Yes, you do take turns, but that's not really compromising. Compromising is coming up with a plan so that everyone is happy. We'd have to talk it out and compromise where we'd work out a plan to do something.
Alex: Like we'd agree to do something – like vote?	
	Mrs. Kerry: Yes. We could vote to see if you want the order of your names changed on the board, but that doesn't really make any sense for right now, and it would take away from you guys talking to each other.
Will: Hey guys, I've got a question. Alex: Like voting on something.	
	Mrs. Kerry: Yes.
Will: Hey guys, I've got a question. How do you say Kindle Fire right? Alex: It's like Kindle, you know how it's fire like camp fire. That's how you do. Will: A regular Kindle is a Kindle Fire? Alex and Cody: Yeah. Will: My aunt. I call her Aunt Sharon. It's going to cost $200 dollars. Cody: Wow. Will: She's going to spend that money to buy me that one Kindle. Cody: I have a real phone today. Will: Can you call people with it? Cody: No. Will: Does it have games on it? Cody: Yeah. Will: Hey guys …	
	Mrs. Kerry: Okay, I'm going to limit you from saying "hey guys." You don't want to do it over and over again in a conversation. You would just want to do it once or twice. You're going to have their attention. They are right here.
Will: So uh. There's this game where everything looks like Minecraft.	
	Mrs. Kerry: Are they interested?

CHAPTER 6: STRATEGIES FOR TEACHING THE CONVERSATION FRAMEWORK

Students' Conversation	Adult Prompts
Alex: Yeah I am. Cody: Not me.	
	Mrs. Kerry: Have you thought about whether or not they are interested?
Will: No, sorry. Alex: That's okay, I'm interested. Will: Hey, Cody (person who said he wasn't interested), have you ever played the game Survival Craft? Cody: Uh, I played Zombie Crypt where there's zombies. Will: Hey guys ...	
	Mrs. Kerry: Okay, wait. You're about to change the topic from what he just said?
Will: Yes, ma'am.	
	Mrs. Kerry: Let's not do that right now.

If tracking the conversation using the Tally Mark Chart for each question (Q), story (S), and comment (C), the chart would look like this:

	Q	S	C
Will	ⅠⅠⅠⅠ ⅠⅠ	Ⅰ	ⅠⅠⅠⅠ
Alex	Ⅰ		ⅠⅠⅠⅠ ⅠⅠ
Cody	ⅠⅠ	Ⅰ	ⅠⅠⅠⅠ

Bridge Visual

The Bridge Visual (see Appendix Q) is a visual support for Step 3 of the Conversation Framework. This tool allows a group of students to see the different ways by which they can change the flow of the conversation. This is important because it shows that you can change the conversation to multiple different topics and aids in developing flexibility of thought. The goal is for the students to be able to fill out the visual without assistance. Please refer to Chapter 4 for an explanation of Bridging the Topic.

NOTE: The Bridge Visual is not used during Steps 1 or 2 of the Conversation Framework.

During Step 3

1. Start by stating a phrase, sentence, or short story and writing the topic on the top line of the Bridge Visual (see Appendix Q). The starting phrase, sentence, or short story should be simple because the next concept will be difficult. (When teaching this step at first, *do not* use a fast-paced audio recording unless the recording is simple and straightforward. Fast-paced audio recordings can be helpful once the student understands how to bridge the topic and can appropriately bridge it in natural conversation.)

TALK WITH ME

2. Say, "How can you bridge this topic to something else?" Prompt the students to look at their Conversation Topics List for ideas. If the students cannot come up with anything, have them look at each of the items on the Conversation Topics List (see Appendix C or D) or other Bridge Visuals (see Appendix Q). While reviewing the items, you can say, "Could you bridge it to (*name topic from list*)?" starting with the top-left item. Go down each topic and say, "Could this be bridged to people/lives?" Continue to go through all the conversation topics like this with the student giving a "yes" or "no" response.

3. Write each of the "yes" ideas under one of the vertical lines. Continue until each vertical line is used. These are now related topics that can be used to take the conversation in an alternate direction without making a drastic topic change.

4. Encourage correct responses and redirect incorrect responses by asking what else it could be. Only write correct responses on the chart. If the students cannot come up with anything other than the first topic or can only come up with topics that are similar, say that their response is not correct. Unless they become stuck on one idea, do not tell the students that they are incorrect to avoid discouraging them.

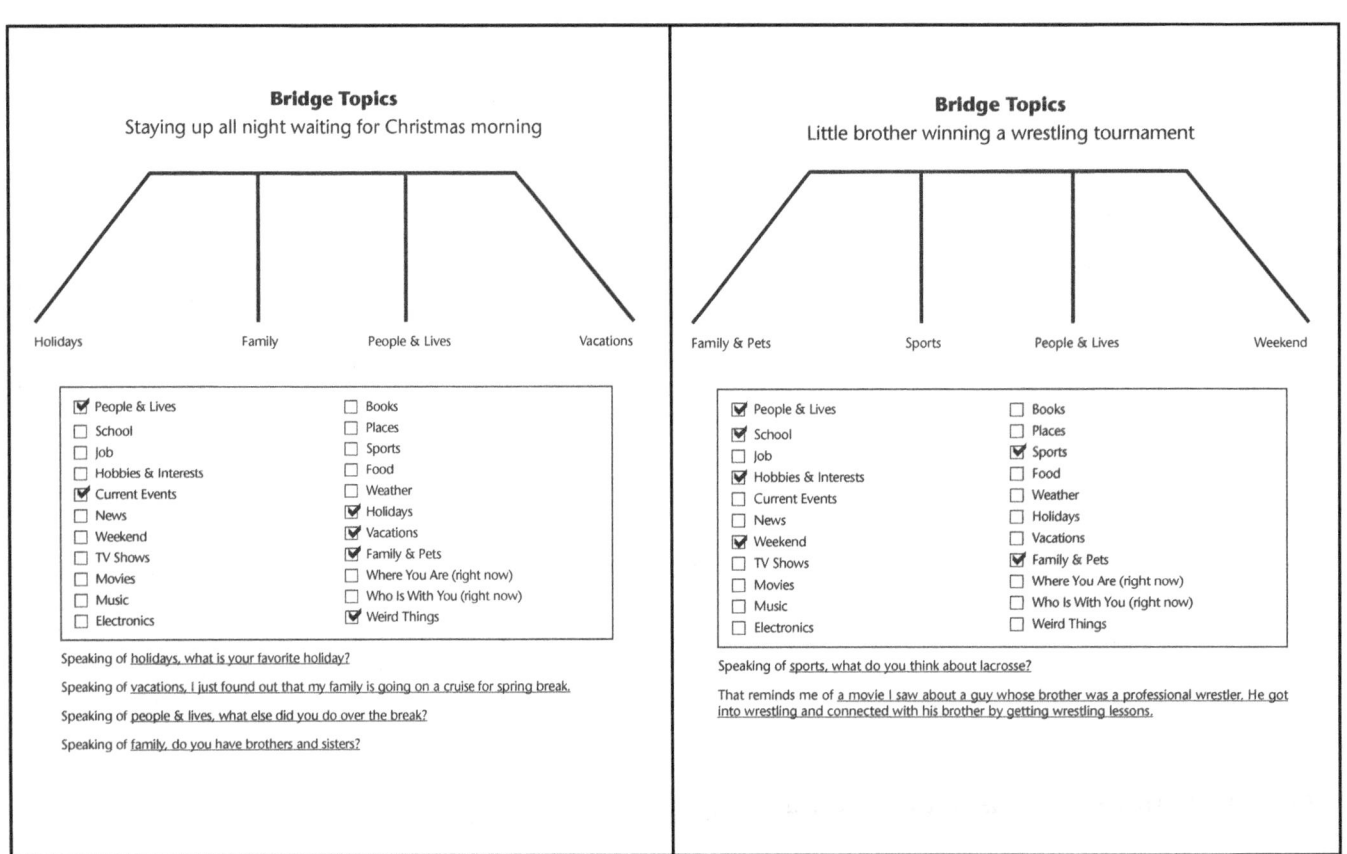

134

CHAPTER 6: STRATEGIES FOR TEACHING THE CONVERSATION FRAMEWORK

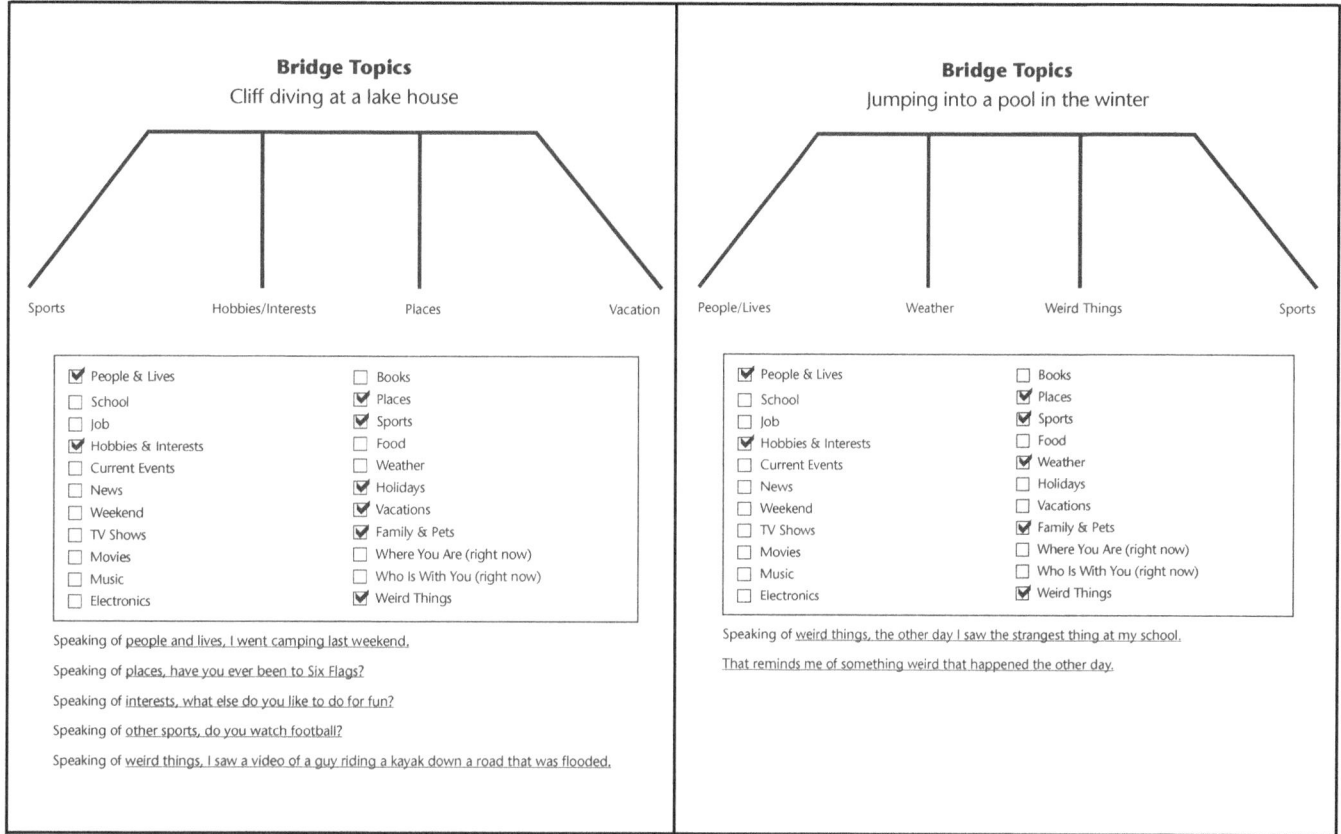

Common Category Chart

The Common Category Chart (see Appendix R) is a visual support for Step 3 of the Conversation Framework. This tool helps a student or group of students to visualize how they could get from a current topic to another appropriate topic. The goal is for the students to be able to fill out the visual without assistance. Please refer to Chapter 4 for an explanation of Bridging the Topic. When using the Common Category Chart, many students with HF-ASD are quick to use two given topics in one sentence without a seamless transition between them. For example, they may try to join the two topics together in one sentence without attention to the flow because identifying the common category is difficult for them.

1. Start by explaining to the student that you will give two topics and that the goal is to smoothly transition the conversation from the first topic to the second topic.
2. Give a starting topic and a topic to transition to.
3. Have the student use questions, stories, or comments to bridge the topic from the starting topic to the ending topic through common categories.

Transitioning Using Common Categories	
Beach → Washington DC Common Category: Vacations, Places (see Appendix R) Questions or Stories for How You Would Transition From One Topic to the Next: • How often have you gone to the beach? • Where are other places you've been to? • Have you ever been to Washington, DC? Incorrect Transition: • I went to a beach in Washington DC.	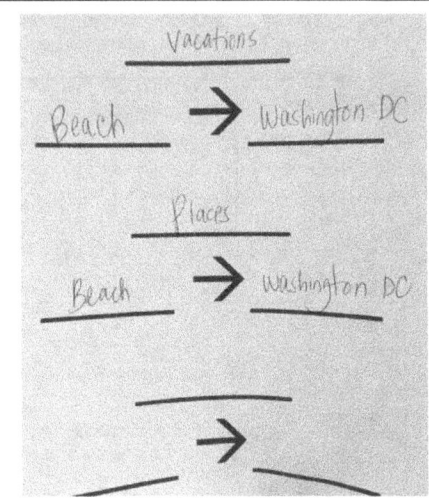
Nook (ebook Reader) → TV Shows Common Category: Electronics, Hobbies & Interests (see Appendix R) Questions or Stories for How You Would Transition From One Topic to the Next: • What do you use it for … books, music, or movies? • Why do you just do books? • So what's your other form of entertainment besides a Nook? • Do you like TV as well? Incorrect Transition: • Do you ever watch tv shows on a Nook?	
Skydiving → Rock of Gibraltar Common Category: People & Lives, Hobbies, Sports (see Appendix R) Questions or Stories for How You Would Transition From One Topic to the Next: • Where do you like to go skydiving? • Do you like any other outdoor sports? • Do you ever go hiking? • Have you ever heard of the Rock of Gibraltar? Incorrect Transition: • Have you ever gone skydiving off the Rock of Gibraltar?	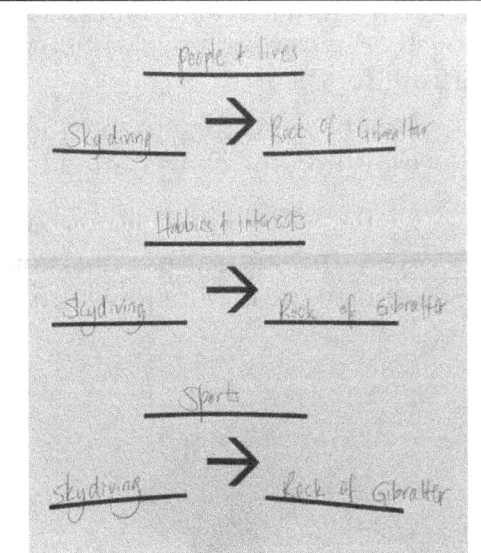

CHAPTER 6: STRATEGIES FOR TEACHING THE CONVERSATION FRAMEWORK

Transition Cards

Transition Cards (see Appendix S) are simple note cards that are used to help a student to visually recognize how conversation categories and topics are connected. This tool is only used during Step 3 of the Conversation Framework. Please refer to Chapter 4 for more information on Bridging the Topic.

During Step 3

1. Make photocopies of the Transition Cards (see Appendix S). Have plenty of blank copies because one card can lead to another and so on.

2. Start by writing the original topic in the center of one of the cards. As the conversation happens, write the details in the blank corners. As the student is learning this transition process, consider using the Transition Cards with labels for "specific" and "general," as this can help the student to know whether the category needs to be condensed or expanded.

3. As the conversation continues, it will flow to another topic. When this happens, write down the new topic on a blank Transition Card.

4. After the conversation, go back over with the student and have him practice arranging the cards to match the flow of the conversation.

5. Once the student is able to arrange the Transition Cards to match the flow of the conversation, explain that you will give him two topics and that he needs to transition the topic from the first topic to the last.

6. Have him write out the starting and ending topic on two Transition Cards.

7. Have him fill in other Transition Cards to smoothly change the starting topic to the ending topic. Each corner that is touching should have the same word(s) written.

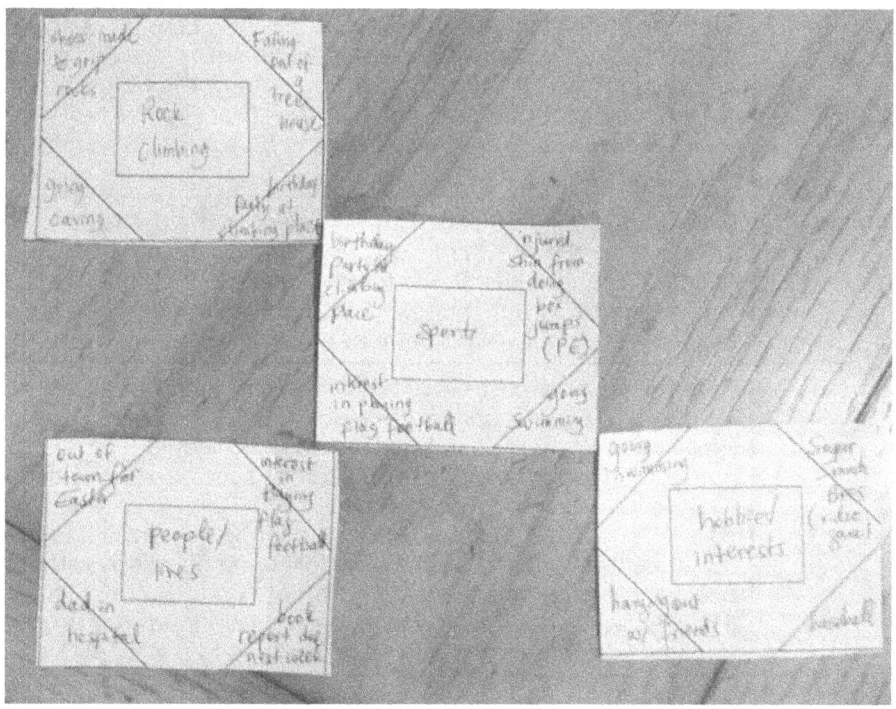

DRILLS

For many with HF-ASD, becoming proficient at conversation requires drills. Drills help to develop the automaticity and speed that everyday conversation demands. Table 6.1 provides simple strategies that can be used for each step of the Conversation Framework. Please refer to Chapter 4 for descriptions of each step within the Conversation Framework, as needed.

Table 6.1
Strategies for Teaching the Steps of the Conversation Framework

Conversation Framework Step	Description
Step 1: Identifying the Topic	**Memorize the Conversation Topics** – Give the students the Conversation Topics List (see Appendices C and D) to memorize for a 2-5 minutes during the session or to take home to memorize before the next session.
Step 1: Identifying the Topic	**How Many** – Ask the students to recall as many general conversation topics from the Conversation Topics List (see Appendices C and D) from memory as possible. Afterwards, use the Conversation Topics List as a teaching tool to learn additional conversation topics that were not said aloud.
Step 1: Identifying the Topic	**Fast-Paced Audio Recordings** – Explain to the student that he will be working on identifying the topic. Explain that you will point to the student, who should then quickly guess the topic. Once the expectations have been explained, play part of a fast-paced audio recording (see pages 124-129). As soon as the topic is identifiable, push "pause" and point to the student. If appropriate, use the Conversation Topics visual to support the student is labeling general topics. Record all responses and hesitation time for data collection.
Step 1: Identifying the Topic	**Main Topic** – Tell a story. Make sure the story consists of at least five sentences. Alternatively, you can use fast-paced audio recordings to simulate a conversation. The student's task is to select three topics from the Conversation Topics List that are appropriate for the conversation. Keep data on the hesitation time for each topic. The end goal is for the student to be able to give three topics with under 2 seconds of hesitation time.
Step 2: Asking Questions	**Give 3** – Make statements such as "I went to the zoo today," "Christmas is my favorite time of year," "I'm ready for school to be out," or "I just got back from Atlanta." The students' task is to ask three follow-up questions. Keep data on hesitation between a statement and each follow-up question. The goal is for students to ask all three follow-up questions without hesitation.
Step 2: Asking Questions	**Fast-Paced Audio Recordings** – Explain to the students that they will be working on asking follow-up questions about what the person on the audio just said. Explain that you will point to a student, who should then quickly ask a follow-up question on topic. Once the expectations have been explained, play part of a fast-paced audio recording (see pages 124-129). As soon as the topic is identifiable, push "pause" and point to a student. Refrain from answering the question if the student is trying to ask multiple follow-up questions without hesitation time, but point to the student again to prompt him to ask another follow-up question. If the student is not asking a follow-up question, prompt by saying, "Follow-up question." Record all responses and hesitation time for data collection.

CHAPTER 6: STRATEGIES FOR TEACHING THE CONVERSATION FRAMEWORK

Conversation Framework Step	Description
Step 2: Asking Questions	**Hot Seat** – Have two students sit in chairs in front of an audience (peers who are not in the hot seat). Give them a set amount of time (usually 1-2 minutes) to try to get the other person to talk. At the end, the audience votes on who was best at asking questions to the other person. The winner gets to stay in the hot seat and choose another opponent.
Step 2: Asking Questions	**Question Game** – This is typically a student favorite! Have one student start the game by asking a question. Instead of answering the question, the next student must turn to someone else and ask a question. Players are "out" if they (a) answer the question instead of passing it on to somebody else, (b) ask the same question of the next person, or (c) hesitate for 2 seconds or more before asking a question of the next person.
Step 2: Asking Questions	**Advanced Question Game** – Play this the same way as the Question Game; however, this time determine a topic that everyone must talk about. In addition to regular outs, players are out if they ask a question off-topic. Predetermined topics can be easy or hard, depending on the individuals in your group.
Step 2: Asking Questions	**Last One Standing** – Pick a leader for each round who is to make a general statement. Moving clockwise, each player asks a follow-up question based on the statement. If the person hesitates, asks a question off-topic, or cannot think of a question, she is out. Once a follow-up question is asked, the leader points to the next person to ask a follow-up question without answering the question.
Step 2: Telling Stories	**Related Stories** – Allow a student to start by telling a natural story of his choosing. Moving clockwise around the circle, allow everyone a turn telling a story related to the topic of the previous story. The first and the third stories do not have to be on the same topic, but they should be connected because the second story is about the same topic as the other two. The most important thing is that each story is related to some topic within the story right before it. To be successful at this requires that students have to listen to every story to know what the topic is. It also makes it a more natural conversation. NOTE: Only play this game if someone within the group needs practice telling stories of on an appropriate topic or talking on topic. Otherwise, this game will not benefit the students in real-life conversations.
Step 2: Telling Stories	**Story Pop** – Have everyone sit in a circle. Ask one student to start a story. Then say, "Pop." Moving clockwise, the next student is to jump in and tell a related story upon hearing the word *pop*. The students must be listening attentively to know the topic so their story is related to the topic of the previous story.
Step 2: Making Comments	**Fast-Paced Audio Recordings** – Explain to the students that they will be working on making comments about what a person just said and that you will use an audio clip to help. Explain that you will point to a student, who should then quickly make a comment on topic. Emphasize that it will be helpful to really listen carefully to what is being said so the student will know if she needs to make a positive or negative comment, such as "oh no" or "that's exciting." Once the expectations have been explained, play part of a fast-paced audio recording (see pages 124-129). As soon as the topic is identifiable, push "pause" and point to the student. Ask the student to make an appropriate comment. If the student is trying to give multiple comments, quickly point to the student again to prompt him to make another comment. If the student is not making a comment, you may prompt by saying, "Make a comment." Record all responses and hesitation time for data collection.

Conversation Framework Step	Description
Step 2: Making Comments	**Give 3** – Tell the students that they will be practicing comments. Make a combination of positive and negative statements (e.g., "I just saw the movie that I wanted to see," "My dad is in the hospital," "My dog got hit by a car"). The students' task is to make three appropriate comments. Keep data on hesitation time before each comment. The goal is to say three comments without hesitation.
Step 2: Making Comments (Girls)	**"That Sounds …"** – Many females become disconnected within close relationships if they have difficulty showing emotional understanding during conversation. For this activity, make a statement that would elicit an emotion (e.g., "My brother had to go into the hospital today," "My teacher just had her baby," "I'm so tired of my sister hogging the bathroom in the morning when I need to get ready," or "He does it just to bother me."). Students' task is to say, "That sounds (give an appropriate emotion). Keep data on hesitation time before each emotional response. The goal is to make a comment expressing emotion without hesitation. If "That sounds …" is too formal for a given group of students, use "That's …" *Example:* That sounds … Annoying Frustrating Weird Stressful Exciting Amazing Scary Rude Disappointing Mean Embarrassing Sad Not fair NOTE: This is a valuable skill for males as well; however, it tends to be females who seem to become more isolated or "judged" for lack of this skill.
Step 3: Bridging the Topic	**Bridging Topics** – Provide a starting topic. The starting topic may be determined by something the group was just discussing or topic based on a current event, etc. After the topic is announced, request that students think of as many related conversational categories (topics) as they can. The main point is for students to verbally identify the new topics. This should be done in drill format to increase students' flexibility and planning with regard to generating new conversational topic ideas rather than starting a conversation. The more new and related conversational categories (topics) that can be identified, the better. If students are identifying details of the given topic, visually show them how their response is part of the initial topic and redirecting them to think of something that is related without being the same.
Step 3: Bridging the Topic	**Bridge** – Start students on a certain topic with the understanding that they will need to change topic when you say "bridge." They are to use the tools they have learned to bridge the topic to something related using scripts (e.g., "Speaking of …," "That reminds me of …").

CHAPTER 6: STRATEGIES FOR TEACHING THE CONVERSATION FRAMEWORK

Conversation Framework Step	Description
Step 3: Bridging the Topic	**Bridge Visual** – Provide a starting topic. The starting topic, often given by the group facilitator or therapist, can be determined by something the group was just discussing or a hypothetical topic based on a current event or thought in an individual setting. After the given topic is said, request for the student to think of as many related conversational categories (topics) as they can. The main point is for the student to verbally identify the new topics. This should be done in drill format, to increase the student's flexibility and planning to generate new conversational topic ideas, rather than starting a conversation. The more new and related conversational categories (topics) that can be identified, the better. If the student is identifying details of the given topic, visually show them as a part of the same topic while redirecting them to think of something that is related.
Step 3: Bridging the Topic	**Transition Cards** – Review with the students the nature of the Transition Cards. The middle space is for the main topic of the conversation. The corners are for the details of the conversation. Both the main topic and the details can be specific or general. For example, if a group of students talk about the Star Wars franchise, the main topic would be a general topic of Star Wars. However, if the topic is a specific Star Wars game, then the main topic would be that game which is specific. Have the student listen to a recording of a conversation. Give them a set of Transition Cards (see Appendix S). Have them fill out the specific and general topics for each topic in the recording. Then have them arrange the cards corner-to-corner so that each topic is showing and how the conversation got to the topic. The corner of one card should have the same specific or general topic as the corner of the card it is connected to. The topic in the middle should be different from the topic on any corner and should be different from the previous card. If the middle is the same on both cards, this means that the conversation stayed on the same topic and, therefore, would not require an extra card.

Conversation Example With Prompts

The following example shows how prompts are used within an individual session. Throughout our sessions, we use a combination of verbal and visual prompts. The prompts are used to guide, redirect, refocus, and encourage students.

Age: 17 years old

Gender: Male

Group Size: 1 student (individual session)

Conversational Goals: Andrew – Step 1: Identifying the Topic

Strategy for Teaching the Conversation Framework

Fast-Paced Audio Recording

Student's Responses	Adult Prompts
NOTE: We listened to a 2-minute, 36-second clip (Blake Sims interview/career after playing football at Alabama)	
	Mrs. Kerry: What's the topic?
Andrew: They are talking about a past football player and his championships and what he's done in the past.	
	Mrs. Kerry: Were they talking about anything else?

TALK WITH ME

Student's Responses	Adult Prompts
Andrew: That's pretty much what I can remember. Oh yea, plus about his interview he was giving.	
	Mrs. Kerry: What was the main topic of that?
Andrew: The interview?	
	Mrs. Kerry: Yes.
Andrew: Sort of why he didn't give the interview much and why he didn't talk much. They were concerned about why he didn't say anything during the interview.	
	Mrs. Kerry: Great! Keep this conversation going.
Andrew: Oh, if I jumped into this conversation?	
	Mrs. Kerry: Yes, but remember just to jump in without saying that.
Andrew: So, what was this guy's name?	
	Mrs. Kerry: Blake Sims is who they were talking about.
Andrew: Which school did he go to?	
	Mrs. Kerry: He played quarterback at Alabama.
Andrew: Oh right. Does he have a family?	
	Mrs. Kerry: Is that the most obvious question to ask me based on what you said the main topic was from the recording?
Andrew: No. What is your favorite thing about him? What do you like most about it?	
	Mrs. Kerry: I probably wouldn't ask that either. You said the topic was about him winning championships and the interview where he didn't talk much.
Andrew: Why didn't he say much during the interview?	
	Mrs. Kerry: I don't know because I didn't listen to the interview, but they were saying that he sounded tired during the interview.
Andrew: What kind of career do you think he is going to get?	
	Mrs. Kerry: Some guys who have had success in football go on to do talk radio and things like that. I don't actually know what he'll do. Now bridge that to another topic.
Andrew: Speaking of jobs, I heard one of my friends works at Carmike Cinemas. He got the job a couple of weeks ago.	
	Mrs. Kerry: Keep it going.
Andrew: Plus, he gets pretty good discounts.	

CHAPTER 6: STRATEGIES FOR TEACHING THE CONVERSATION FRAMEWORK

Student's Responses	Adult Prompts
	Mrs. Kerry: How can you include me in the conversation?
Andrew: What is your favorite thing to do in the theater – eat popcorn or watch a movie, 2D or 3D, ya know.	
	Mrs. Kerry: I wouldn't ask about my favorite thing to do in the theater. What is the most obvious question that you can ask about that topic?
Andrew: What kind of job would you like to get?	
	Mrs. Kerry: Do I already have a job?
Andrew: Yes.	
	Mrs. Kerry: Going back to my favorite thing to do in the theater, what's a more obvious question you can ask about that?
Andrew: What type of food do you like in the theater? Do you like going to the movies?	
	Mrs. Kerry: You can ask me if I like going to the movies, and yes I do. Keep it going.
Andrew: Which movie is your favorite?	
	Mrs. Kerry: Is there a better question you can ask?
Andrew: Do you know any movies coming soon?	
	Mrs. Kerry: Perfect! Or you can ask about movies out now, which would go under the conversation category of movies or what else?
Andrew: What type of movies do you like?	
	Mrs. Kerry: No like what type of conversation categories would "Do you know of any movies coming soon?" be under? It would be under movies, people/lives, what else …
Andrew: What other question I come up with?	
	Mrs. Kerry: Now remember that sheet that you memorized? Let me get it out.
Andrew: Oh right! *Action*.	
	Mrs. Kerry: *Action* is not a category from our conversation categories sheet.
Andrew: Friends … jobs	
	Mrs. Kerry: What else?
Andrew: Current events … people …TV	
	Mrs. Kerry: TV isn't really a category for movies. You need to know the other related categories to help you bridge the topic to something else.

> **Teaching How to Form a Question**
> When teaching preschool students or students who don't know how to form a question, one person should tell a story, and everybody else has to ask one question or make one comment about what the person just said.

PROMPTS

A prompt is a reminder or cue signaling a person where to direct his attention. Prompts can be verbal or visual. Too often, teachers are quick to break down a conversation for someone by saying, "They are talking about (*fill in subject here*)," and we automatically give someone the topic through our prompt. Although that is a polite gesture, this type of prompting does not allow the student to think for himself and, thus, becomes a barrier to independence.

When learning how to correctly identify the topic, students may need to listen to the conversation many times, which is why a fast-paced audio recording can be a valuable tool. If a fast-paced audio recording is not available or appropriate for the conversation at hand, prompt the student to say, "Can you repeat that?" or "What did you say?" The scripts for requesting that someone repeat what they said will vary depending on what is polite in your home, school, or community.

Prompts are necessary throughout every step of the Conversation Framework. However, in order to help students achieve independence with conversation, it is important that prompts are given in a way that can be faded easily. To do this, choose a verbal, visual, gesture, or behavior prompt as necessary to teach the skill without doing the entire skill for the student. For example, you may prompt your student to ask a follow-up question or tell a related story, but do not create the follow-up question or related story for him. Start with very simplistic prompts and only provide examples, carrier phrases, or scripting when necessary because simpler prompts are not effective. If the student requires verbal prompts, eventually fade the verbal prompts to gesture prompts, which are typically easier to fade. The number of prompts will eventually need to diminish for the student to participate in conversation independently. Once the student begins to understand what is being taught, start reducing the number of prompts until no prompts are necessary for the student to do the skill on his own. Practice the skill again and again. Using repeated practice (see Chapter 2) often allows for prompts to be faded because the student has a better understanding of what is being asked.

Keep in mind that a student has not mastered a step within the Conversation Framework if he is still requiring prompts to do it. Mastery is achieved when a step is done independently. Only prompt what your student needs. Do not overprompt. Many adults prompt out of a desire to teach or compensate for awkward pauses while waiting for somebody to talk. The Conversation Framework teaches the skills necessary to engage successfully in conversations; teachers need to trust the step-by-step process with the understanding that the ability to think of what to say will increase and the hesitation time will decrease with practice. *A prompt-dependent student is only prompt dependent because of the prompts he is receiving.*

Verbal Prompts

Verbal prompts are prompts that are presented orally to assist students in learning the material presented. Verbal prompts can include oral reminders whispered individually or stated out loud individually or in a group setting.

CHAPTER 6: STRATEGIES FOR TEACHING THE CONVERSATION FRAMEWORK

Carrier phrases (see Appendices L and M) are the first word or words in a sentence whereby the adult starts and the student completes the sentence. Carrier phrases can be used as a verbal prompt. Students should repeat the carrier phrase before completing the sentence.

Table 6.2 presents examples of verbal prompts and their purpose.

Table 6.2
Verbal Prompts Examples Given by Adult

Embedded Skills	
Verbal Prompt	**Purpose of Prompt**
Say, "It's important for you to recognize being bored, but don't show that you're bored."	This may be appropriate in a group setting when you are embedding the skill of body language.
Say, "Just jump in."	This may be appropriate in a group setting when you are embedding the skill of timing.
Say, "Wait for a pause."	This may be appropriate in a group setting when you are embedding the skill of timing.
Say, "If you notice someone starts talking, stop talking."	This may be appropriate in a group setting when you are embedding the skill of timing and active listening.
Say, "Say, 'What did you just say?'"	This is generally used to promote active listening and to ensure that a student understands the topic.
Say, "Say, 'Please say it one more time.'"	If a student is unable to verbalize what someone said, this is generally stated to the conversation partner so he will repeat what he said one more time to allow the student another chance for to identify the topic correctly.
Say, "Say, 'We were just talking about …'"	This is generally used to include someone in the conversation if they are just entering the room or the conversation.
Say, "Take a bite, stop and talk."	This may be appropriate in an individual or group setting when you are embedding the skill of timing. It teaches a student how to talk while eating.
Say, "That's really formal."	This may be appropriate to draw attention to the student's use of formal vs. informal language.
Identifying the Topic	
Prompt	**Purpose of Prompt**
Whisper, "What is the topic?"	This may be appropriate for students who embarrass easily.
Say aloud, "What is the topic?"	This may be appropriate when several students within the social group are learning to identify the topic.
Pause the audio recording and say, "What is the topic?"	This may be appropriate for students who embarrass easily, students who need additional time to process the topic, or students who often misidentify the topic and need more practice.
Explain: "The topic is like the main point – it's what the whole thing is about."	This may be appropriate for students who are learning the concept of identifying the topic.

145

TALK WITH ME

Balancing the Conversation	
Prompt	**Purpose of Prompt**
Say, "Is your conversation balanced?"	This may be appropriate for students who are learning the concept of balancing the conversation.
Say, "What do you need to do more of?"	This may be appropriate for students who are learning the concept of balancing the conversation.
Say, "What do you need to do to make the conversation balanced?"	This may be appropriate for students who are learning the concept of balancing the conversation.
Say, "What makes this conversation balanced?"	This may be appropriate for students who are learning the concept of balancing the conversation.
Say, "What makes this conversation unbalanced?"	This may be appropriate for students who are learning the concept of balancing the conversation.
Say, "Balancing the conversation is trying to get something in each square – you want to try to ask questions, tell stories, and make comments."	This may be appropriate for students who are learning the concept of balancing the conversation.
Say, "Remember only one person talks at a time."	This may be appropriate when one student interrupts when another is speaking.
Asking Questions	
Prompt	**Purpose of Prompt**
Whisper, "What's your follow-up question?"	This may be appropriate for students who embarrass easily.
Say, "_____ (name), what were you going to ask?"	This may be appropriate when several students within the social group are learning to ask questions.
Say, "How would you include them in the conversation?"	This helpful to remind a student to ask a question.
Say, "Say, 'What about you?'"	This may be appropriate to prompt a student to remember to ask about someone else.
Say, "Try hard to remember what it is that he's talking about. It's important in conversation."	This reminds the student of his task when another person is speaking in a conversation.
Telling Stories	
Prompt	**Purpose of Prompt**
Whisper, "Tell a related story."	This may be appropriate for students who embarrass easily.
Say, "_____ (name), what story were you going to tell on topic?"	This may be appropriate when several students within the social group are learning to tell stories.
Say, "What does their story make you think of? What is a related story you could tell about *your* experience?"	This may be appropriate when several students within the social group are learning to tell stories.
Say, "Are they interested?"	This reminds a student to notice the response of others to his story.
Say, "I …"	Using carrier phrases may be appropriate to support an individual or group in starting to tell a story.
Say, "My …"	Using carrier phrases may be appropriate to support an individual or group in starting to tell a story.

CHAPTER 6: STRATEGIES FOR TEACHING THE CONVERSATION FRAMEWORK

Making Comments	
Prompt	**Purpose of Prompt**
Whisper, "Make a comment."	This may be appropriate for students who embarrass easily.
Say, "_____ (name), what comment can you make to show interest?"	This may be appropriate when several students within the social group are learning to make comments.
Say, "It's better to say 'I've never seen it' or 'I've never heard of it' than to say nothing."	This may be appropriate when several students within the social group are learning to make comments.
Say, "That sounds …"	This may be appropriate when a female within the social group is learning to make comments.
Say, "Make a comment and get back on topic."	This may be appropriate when several students within the social group are making comments that lead the conversation to a light topic because of making back-to-back light comments.
Bridging the Topic	
Prompt	**Purpose of Prompt**
Say, "That's a specific topic, so we need to generalize that out."	This may help when a student is talking about specifics related to a topic rather than changing the topic to a related general topic.
Say, "What will happen is that it will bridge into something else."	This may help when a student is learning to use a common category.
Say, "What you need to do is draw an arrow which will lead you into this card."	This may help a student see how topics connect using the Transition Cards.
Say, "That reminds me of …"	Using carrier phrases may be appropriate to support an individual or group in bridging the topic to a new related topic.
Say, "Speaking of …"	Using carrier phrases may be appropriate to support an individual or group in bridging the topic to a new related topic.

Visual Prompts

Visual prompts are prompts that are presented visually to assist the student in learning the material presented. Visual prompts can include reminders written on a dry-erase board, note cards, or a sheet of paper. Visual prompts are appropriate for students who need a visual reminder within the group context or to identify the topic. Table 6.3 shows examples of visual prompts related to the Conversation Framework.

Table 6.3
Examples of Visual Prompts Related to the Conversation Framework

---

IDENTIFY THE TOPIC

TOPIC _____

ASK QUESTIONS

Follow-Up Question

Ask about the OTHER person

"What about YOU?"

ASK QUESTIONS
Who __?
What __?
When __?
Where __?
Do you __?

TELLING STORIES
1.
2.
3.
4.
5.

One time …

I …

First,…

Then,…

Last,…

MAKING COMMENTS
"Cool"
"Awesome"
"I've never seen it"

BRIDGING THE TOPIC
That reminds me of …
Speaking of …
This is a little off-topic, but …
That sort of relates to …
Speaking of which …
By the way …

CHAPTER 6: STRATEGIES FOR TEACHING THE CONVERSATION FRAMEWORK

Gesture Prompts

Gesture prompts can be effective in teaching concepts such as volume, longer stories, and turn taking. Once a gesture has been agreed upon between the student and adult, gesture prompts can be given from further distances for a variety of purposes rather than being limited to prompting in close proximity.

The following are examples of gesture prompts:

- Point to the student when a pause has occurred in the conversation to signal good timing to "jump into" the conversation.
- Wave hand to symbolize "keep going" when a student is working on telling a longer story.
- Point to a student to symbolize that it is his turn.
- Point to yourself to symbolize that the student is to ask you a question.
- Point to a peer in the group or activity to symbolize that the student is to ask that person a question or include the person in the conversation.
- Hold up your pointer and middle finger in the shape of a "V" to symbolize voice volume, whether the gesture prompt has been pre-determined to reference turning up her volume or lowering her volume. Some students prefer the "V" to be upside down with the pointer and middle finger pointing to the ground when symbolizing to lower their volume.

Behavior Prompts

In some instances, minor behaviors often rooted in inflexibility or lack of awareness can impede the conversation between people. For example, Brian is a fourth-grade student with HF-ASD who often corrects others for what he perceives to be an incorrect pronunciation of a word. Rather than letting it go if others do not comply with his suggestions, Brian's frustration tends to escalate to the point that he needs to leave the room, often slamming the door behind him. This is a situation that may benefit from a behavior prompt such as preteaching (e.g., "Would you rather be arguing or talking about your favorite topic?," "Does the pronunciation of the word make for an interesting conversation?"). Preteaching flexibility like this can equip Brian to be more successful in the practice environment.

Verbal, visual, and gesture prompts may also be helpful to redirect behavior depending on the situation. Diffusing negative behaviors allows for the development of conversation skills discussed within the Conversation Framework that will later generalize to a wide range of settings when learned.

Minor behaviors that can have a major impact on conversation include using formal language when starting a conversation, asking for permission to start a topic in the middle of an informal conversation, talking about an uninteresting and irrelevant detail on a special interest, and asking others what they want to talk about. If you have a student who tends to start a conversation very formally (e.g., "What do you want to talk about," "Let's talk about spring break"), please refer to the prompts in Table 6.4.

Table 6.4
Prompts for Specific Conversation Behaviors

Prompt	Purpose of Prompt
Say, "You wouldn't want to say, "I'll start the conversation, just start it."	A verbal prompt may be beneficial to redirect a student from saying something formal to having a more natural conversation with others.
Say, "You don't have to explain it – just say it."	A verbal prompt may be beneficial to redirect a student from saying something formal to having a more natural conversation with others.
Say, "You don't have to plan it – Just say what you were going to say."	A verbal prompt may be beneficial to redirect a student from saying something formal to having a more natural conversation with others.
Say, "Just decide what you're going to talk about and start talking about it."	A verbal prompt may be beneficial to redirect a student from saying something formal to having a more natural conversation with others.
Say, "Does ___ make for an interesting conversation?"	A verbal prompt may be beneficial to redirect a student to consider whether or not what he intends to say will make an interesting conversation.
~~What do you want to talk about?~~	A visual prompt with a phrase crossed out may help an individual with HF-ASD see that the phrase is not appropriate for starting a conversation.
~~Alright I'll tell you about ...~~	A visual prompt with a phrase crossed out may help an individual with HF-ASD see that the phrase is not appropriate for starting a conversation. It's often paired with a verbal prompt of "Just say it."
~~Hey guys~~	A visual prompt with a phrase crossed out may help an individual with HF-ASD see that she is saying something too many times or the situation is not appropriate for getting somebody's attention.
~~Let's talk about ...~~	A visual prompt with a phrase crossed out may help an individual with HF-ASD see that the phrase is not appropriate for starting a conversation. It's often paired with a verbal prompt of "Just say what you were going to say."
~~You go.~~	A visual prompt with a phrase crossed out may help an individual with HF-ASD see that the phrase is not appropriate for starting a conversation. Pair the visual with a verbal or visual prompt of what the student can say instead (e.g., "I heard ...," "Have you ...?"). It's often paired with a verbal prompt of "Just say what you were going to say."
~~I'll start the conversation.~~	A visual prompt with a phrase crossed out may help an individual with HF-ASD see that the phrase is not appropriate for starting a conversation. Pair the visual with a verbal or visual prompt of what the student can say instead (e.g., "I heard ...," "Have you ...?"). It's often paired with a verbal prompt of "Just say what you were going to say."
Say, "You don't have to raise your hand, just say it."	A verbal prompt may be beneficial to redirect a student from raising his hand to contribute to a conversation in an informal setting.
Say, "Would you rather be arguing or talking about ___?"	A verbal prompt may be beneficial to redirect the focus of the conversation from a minor detail to a common interest or something both people want to discuss. This is often related to items such as the pronunciation of a word and other areas where students with HF-ASD show inflexibility.
Say, "We were just talking about ..."	When someone walks into the room, prompt someone to say, "We were just talking about ..." It is a script that becomes automatic when someone enters the room or conversation. This script helps to automatically include the other person into the conversation.

CHAPTER 6: STRATEGIES FOR TEACHING THE CONVERSATION FRAMEWORK

If you have a student who tends to ask questions to which he or she already knows the answer to or who is off topic, please refer to the prompts in Table 6.5.

Table 6.5
Prompts for Repetitive Questions

Prompt	Purpose of Prompt
Say, "Do you know the answer to that question? (If so, say, "That's not a good question. Ask another question to get an answer that you do not already know.")	A verbal prompt may be beneficial to redirect a student from asking a question to which he already knows the answer to a question that he is curious about and to which he wants to know the answer.
Ask, "Is that on-topic?"	Sometimes the question is off-topic, so this redirects the conversation.
Say, "Do not ask questions you know the answer to."	A verbal prompt may be beneficial to redirect a student from asking a question to which he already knows the answer to a question that he is curious about and to which he wants to know the answer.

A group of 13- to 16-year-old male students were having conversation within their group. One of the students suddenly asked the group facilitator if she liked Luke Bryan. Rather than answering his question, she redirected him to ask the male peers. The conversation is summarized in Table 6.6.

Table 6.6
Example of Redirecting a Student

Students' Conversation	Adult Prompts
Peer 1: I don't like those new artists. I like Tim McGraw, Hank Williams. Peer 2: I like Luke Bryan. Do you like him?	
	Mrs. Kerry: Ask them; don't ask me.
Peer 2: What other music do you like besides country? Peer 3: I like rock n roll – definitely like Elvis and the Beatles. Peer 2: What's your favorite music? Peer 4: I like Toby Mac. Peer 2: What's the type of music you like? Peer 5: I really like Christian music the best. Peer 4: What kind of music do you like? Peer 6: I like classic rock. Peer 2: Do you like rap? Rap is not music to me. Peer 3: I like some rap, but not all of it. Peer 6: Me, too.	

CHAPTER 7
SETTING IEP GOALS WITHIN THE CONVERSATION FRAMEWORK

It is important to incorporate the Conversation Framework into your student's IEP if the IEP team agrees that conversation skills are relevant to the student's success. The IEP goals presented here are recommendations and ideas that *may* be appropriate for your student. With your IEP team, please discuss the most important needs for your student to make sure his or her immediate needs are being addressed. The IEP goals should be matched to the conversation step that your student is on, which can be determined through the use of the assessments in Chapter 5.

Please keep in mind that the Conversation Framework is a methodical teaching tool that requires mastery of a given step before moving on to the next. IEP goal mastery criteria should be based on professional judgment and may include the use of prompts (e.g., 1, 2, 3, and/or type of prompt, such as a gestural, visual, or verbal prompt), settings (i.e., structured or unstructured), or time period (e.g., within a 4-week period, within a 9-week period).

Before writing an IEP goal into the student's IEP, please ensure that you are developing a goal that is relevant to the student's needs. Chapter 5 provides assessment tools that are helpful for determining which step of the Conversation Framework should be taught first.

IEP GOALS FOR STEP 1 – IDENTIFYING THE TOPIC

Goal: Student will show proficiency in correctly identifying the topic being discussed.

- Within 2 seconds, student will correctly identify the topic in fast-paced audio recordings within a structured setting (assign criteria for mastery).

- Within 2 seconds, student will correctly identify the topic using media (movie, TV show, video recording) within structured setting (assign criteria for mastery).

- Within 2 seconds, student will correctly identify the topic during natural conversations within a structured setting using no more than one visual prompt (assign criteria for mastery).

- Within 2 seconds, student will correctly identify the topic during natural conversations within a structured setting using no more than one verbal prompt (assign criteria for mastery).

- Within 2 seconds, student will correctly identify the topic during natural conversations within a structured setting without prompts (assign criteria for mastery).

- Within 2 seconds, student will correctly identify the topic during natural conversations within unstructured settings (assign criteria for mastery).

- Within 2 seconds, student will correctly identify the weight of the topic (i.e., light, medium, heavy) (assign criteria for mastery).

IEP GOALS FOR STEP 2 – BALANCING THE CONVERSATION USING QUESTIONS, STORIES, & COMMENTS WITHIN 0-2 SECONDS

Goal: Student will show proficiency in balancing questions, stories, and comments in natural conversation settings (assign criteria for mastery).

Goal: Student will show proficiency in balancing questions, stories, and comments in structured conversation settings (assign criteria for mastery).

- Student will ask three follow-up questions on one topic each within 0-2 seconds with one verbal prompt ("Ask a follow-up question") (assign criteria for mastery).

- Student will ask three follow-up questions on one topic each within 0-2 seconds with one gesture prompt to ask a follow-up question (assign criteria for mastery).

- After listening to a fast-paced audio recording, student will ask at least one follow-up question within 0-2 seconds with one verbal or gesture prompt (assign criteria for mastery).

- During a slow-paced conversation in a structured setting, student will ask at least one follow-up question within 0-2 seconds with one verbal or gesture prompt (assign criteria for mastery).

- During a fast-paced conversation in a structured setting, student will ask at least one follow-up question within 0-2 seconds with one verbal or gesture prompt (assign criteria for mastery).

- In a natural conversation with peers, student will ask at least one follow-up question within 0-2 seconds with one verbal or gesture prompt (assign criteria for mastery).

- In a natural conversation with peers, student will spontaneously ask at least one follow-up question within 0-2 seconds (assign criteria for mastery).

- Student will spontaneously ask follow up question within 0-2 seconds (assign criteria for mastery).

- When presented with a random comment, student will articulate three follow-up questions on topic (assign criteria for mastery).

- Student will build fluency of asking questions within 0-2 seconds hesitation time (assign criteria for mastery).

CHAPTER 7: SETTING IEP GOALS WITHIN THE CONVERSATION FRAMEWORK

- After hearing a comment or story, student will tell a related story on a similar topic including at least three consecutive sentences with gesture prompts (assign criteria for mastery).

- After hearing a comment or story, student will spontaneously tell a related story on a similar topic including at least three consecutive sentences without prompts (assign criteria for mastery).

- After hearing a comment or story, student will tell a related story on a similar topic including at least four consecutive sentences with gesture prompts (assign criteria for mastery).

- After hearing a comment or story, student will spontaneously tell a related story on a similar topic including at least four consecutive sentences without prompts (assign criteria for mastery).

- After hearing a comment or story, student will tell a related story on a similar topic including at least five consecutive sentences with gesture prompts (assign criteria for mastery).

- After hearing a comment or story, student will spontaneously tell a related story on a similar topic including at least five consecutive sentences without prompts (assign criteria for mastery).

- After hearing a light story, student will make a comment with appropriate inflection of voice (assign criteria for mastery).

- After hearing a light story, student will make a comment using appropriate body language to mirror the conversation partners (e.g., smiling, leaning in, happy) (assign criteria for mastery).

- After hearing a medium story, student will make a comment on topic (assign criteria for mastery).

- After hearing a heavy story, student will make a comment with appropriate inflection of voice to show an empathetic response (assign criteria for mastery).

- Student will balance components of a conversation in a slow-paced conversation (assign criteria for mastery).

- Student will balance components of a conversation in a slow-paced conversation with one conversational partner (assign criteria for mastery).

- Student will balance components of a conversation in a slow-paced conversation in a small group in a structured setting without background noise (assign criteria for mastery).

- Student will balance components of a conversation in a slow-paced conversation in a small group in structured setting with background noise (assign criteria for mastery).

- Student will balance components of a conversation in a slow-paced conversation in a large group in a structured setting without background noise (assign criteria for mastery).

- Student will balance components of a conversation in a slow-paced conversation in a large group in a structured setting with background noise (assign criteria for mastery).

IEP GOALS FOR STEP 3 – BRIDGING THE TOPIC

Goal: Student will show proficiency in bridging topics to three related topics (assign criteria for mastery).

Goal: Student will show proficiency in making smooth transitions between two topics (assign criteria for mastery).

- Given a general conversation topic in a structured setting, student will generate at least one related topic that the conversation can be bridged to (assign criteria for mastery).

- Given a general conversation topic in a structured setting, student will generate at least two related topics that the conversation can be bridged to (assign criteria for mastery).

- Given a general conversation topic in a structured setting, student will generate at least three related topics that the conversation can be bridged to (assign criteria for mastery).

- Given a general conversation topic in a structured setting, student will independently generate at least one related topic that the conversation can be bridged to (assign criteria for mastery).

- Given a general conversation topic in a structured setting, student will independently generate at least two related topics that the conversation can be bridged to (assign criteria for mastery).

- Given a general conversation topic in a structured setting, student will independently generate at least three related topics that the conversation can be bridged to (assign criteria for mastery).

- Given two topics, student will verbalize a general category for how the two topics can be related together using a common category (assign criteria for mastery).

- Given two topics, student will use at least five sentences to conversationally get from one topic to another with no more than three adult prompts (assign criteria for mastery).

- Given two topics, student will use at least five sentences to conversationally get from one topic to another with no more than two adult prompts (assign criteria for mastery).

- Given two topics, student will use at least five sentences to conversationally get from one topic to another with no more than one adult prompts (assign criteria for mastery).

- Given two topics, student will independently use at least five sentences to conversationally get from one topic to another (assign criteria for mastery).

CHAPTER 7: SETTING IEP GOALS WITHIN THE CONVERSATION FRAMEWORK

IEP GOALS FOR EMBEDDED SKILLS

Goal: Student will show proficiency in using embedded skills in conversation (e.g. insert embedded skill from chapter 3 relevant for the student)

- During a structured setting, student will use a sad voice intonation to make a conversation believable with no more than one prompt (assign criteria for mastery).

- During a natural conversation, student will spontaneously use a sad voice intonation to make a conversation believable (assign criteria for mastery).

- During a structured setting, student will use an excited voice intonation to make a conversation believable with no more than one prompt (assign criteria for mastery).

- During a natural conversation, student will spontaneously use an excited voice intonation to make a conversation believable (assign criteria for mastery).

- During a structured setting, student will use a/an (insert emotion) voice intonation to make a conversation believable with no more than one prompt (assign criteria for mastery).

- During a natural conversation, student will spontaneously use a/an (insert emotion) voice intonation to make a conversation believable (assign criteria for mastery).

- Using a fast-paced audio recording, student will recognize interrupting (assign criteria for mastery).

- Student will verbalize important steps to avoid interrupting (i.e., wait for a pause, one person talking at a time, stop talking if you notice someone talking at the same time) (assign criteria for mastery).

- Using a fast-paced audio recording, student will recognize the pauses in conversation as demonstrated with no more than one gesture prompts (assign criteria for mastery).

- Student will wait for a pause in conversation and will immediately join the conversation at the right time (assign criteria for mastery).

- Student will verbalize important steps to good listening behaviors (i.e., look at the person talking, concentrate on what is being said) (assign criteria for mastery).

- Student will verbalize at least three reasons for listening in a conversation (assign criteria for mastery).

- Student will demonstrate good listening behaviors (e.g., eye contact with speaker, nodding head) (assign criteria for mastery).

- Student will use nonverbal body language (e.g., nodding head, glance at the person talking, look at the person talking) to show listening behaviors (assign criteria for mastery).

- Student will mirror body language of conversation partners (assign criteria for mastery).

REFERENCES

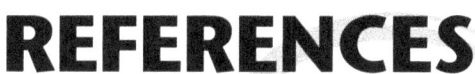

American Psychiatric Association. (2013). *Diagnostic and statistical manual of mental disorders* (5th ed.). Arlington, VA: American Psychiatric Publishing.

Ames, C., & Fletcher-Watson, S. (2010). A review of methods in the study of attention in autism. *Developmental Review, 30*(1), 52-73.

Aspy, G., & Grossman, B. G. (2011). *The Ziggurat Model: A framework for designing comprehensive interventions for individuals with autism and Asperger syndrome.* Shawnee Mission, KS: AAPC Publishing.

Baron-Cohen, S., Wheelwright, S., Hill, J., Raste, Y., & Plumb, I. (2001). The "Reading the Mind in the Eyes" test revised version: A study with normal adults, and adults with Asperger syndrome or high-functioning autism. *Journal of Child Psychology and Psychiatry, 42*(2), 241-251.

Bock, M. A. (1994). Acquisition, maintenance, and generalization of a categorization strategy by children with autism. *Journal of Autism and Developmental Disorders, 24*(1), 39-51.

Bock, M. A. (1999). Sorting laundry categorization strategy application to an authentic learning activity by children with autism. *Focus on Autism and Other Developmental Disabilities, 14*(4), 220-230.

Chin, H. Y., & Bernard-Opitz, V. (2000). Teaching conversational skills to children with autism: Effect on the development of a theory of mind. *Journal of Autism and Developmental Disorders, 30*(6), 569-583.

Church, B. A., Krauss, M. S., Lopata, C., Toomey, J. A., Thomeer, M. L., Coutinho, M. V., ... & Mercado, E. (2010). Atypical categorization in children with high-functioning autism spectrum disorder. *Psychonomic Bulletin & Review, 17*(6), 862-868.

De Rosnay, M., Fink, E., Begeer, S., Slaughter, V., & Peterson, C. (2014). Talking theory of mind talk: Young school-aged children's everyday conversation and understanding of mind and emotion. *Journal of Child Language, 41*(05), 1179-1193.

Diehl, J. J., Bennetto, L., & Young, E. C. (2006). Story recall and narrative coherence of high-functioning children with autism spectrum disorders. *Journal of Abnormal Child Psychology, 34*(1), 83-98.

Flood, A. M., Hare, D. J., & Wallis, P. (2011). An investigation into social information processing in young people with Asperger syndrome. *Autism, 15*(5), 601-624.

Franke, L., & Durbin, C. (2011). *Nurturing narratives: Story-based language intervention for children with language impairments that are complicated by other developmental disabilities such as autism spectrum disorders.* Shawnee Mission, KS: AAPC Publishing.

Gagnon, E., & Myles, B. S. (2016). *The Power Card Strategy 2: Using special interests to motivate children and youth with autism spectrum disorder.* Shawnee Mission, KS: AAPC Publishing.

Goldstein, G., Allen, D. N., Minshew, N. J., Williams, D. L., Volkmar F., Klin, A., & Schultz, R. J. (2008). The structure of intelligence in children and adults with high functioning autism. *Neuropsychology, 22,* 301-312.

Haiman, J. (1998): *Talk is cheap: Sarcasm, alienation, and the evolution of language.* Oxford, England: Oxford University Press.

Hare, D. J., Wood, C., Wastell, S., & Skirrow, P. (2014). Anxiety in Asperger's syndrome: Assessment in real time. *Autism, 19*(5), 542-52.

Holdnack, J., Goldstein, G., & Drozdick, L. (2011). Social perception and WAIS-IV performance in adolescents and adults diagnosed with Asperger's syndrome and autism. *Assessment, 18*(2), 192-200.

Kenworthy, L., Black, D., Wallace, G., Ahluvalia, T., Wagner, A., & Sirian, L. (2005). Disorganization: The forgotten executive dysfunction in high functioning autism spectrum disorders. *Developmental Neuropsychology, 28,* 809-827.

Kleinhans, N., Akshoomoff, N., & Delis, D. C. (2005). Executive functions in autism and Asperger's disorder: Flexibility, fluency, and inhibition. *Developmental Neuropsychology, 27*(3), 379-401.

Kleinhans, N. M., Richards, T., Weaver, K., Johnson, L. C., Greenson, J., Dawson, G., & Aylward, E. (2010). Association between amygdala response to emotional faces and social anxiety in autism spectrum disorders. *Neuropsychologia, 48*(12), 3665-3670.

Koegel, L. K., Koegel, R. L., Green-Hopkins, I., & Barnes, C. C. (2010). Brief report: Question-asking and collateral language acquisition in children with autism. *Journal of Autism and Developmental Disorders, 40*(4), 509-515.

Laugeson, E. A., Frankel, F., Mogil, C., & Dillon, A. R. (2009). Parent-assisted social skills training to improve friendships in teens with autism spectrum disorders. *Journal of Autism and Developmental Disorders, 39*(4), 596-606.

Losh, M., & Capps, L. (2003). Narrative ability in high-functioning children with autism or Asperger's syndrome. *Journal of Autism and Developmental Disorders, 33*(3), 239-251.

Loukusa, S., Leinonen, E., Kuusikko, S., Jussila, K., Mattila, M. L., Ryder, N., ... & Moilanen, I. (2007). Use of context in pragmatic language comprehension by children with Asperger syndrome or high-functioning autism. *Journal of Autism and Developmental Disorders, 37*(6), 1049-1059.

REFERENCES

MacKay, T., Knott, F., & Dunlop, A. W. (2007). Developing social interaction and understanding in individuals with autism spectrum disorder: A groupwork intervention. *Journal of Intellectual and Developmental Disability, 32*(4), 279-290.

Myles, B. S., Aspy, R. (2016). *High-functioning autism and difficult moments: Practical solutions for reducing meltdowns.* Future Horizons.

Myles, B. S., Trautman, M. L., & Schelvan, R. L. (2013). *The hidden curriculum: Practical solutions for understanding unstated rules in social situations* (2nd ed.). Shawnee Mission, KS: AAPC Publishing.

Patel, V. B., Preedy, V. R., & Martin, C. R. (2014). *Comprehensive guide to autism.* New York, NY: Springer.

Peterson, C. C., Garnett, M., Kelly, A., & Attwood, T. (2009). Everyday social and conversation applications of theory-of-mind understanding by children with autism spectrum disorders or typical development. *European Child & Adolescent Psychiatry, 18*(2),105-115.

Rajendran, G., & Mitchell, P. (2006). Text chat as a tool for referential questioning in Asperger syndrome. *Journal of Speech, Language, and Hearing Research, 49*(1), 102-112.

Rehfeldt, R. A., Dillen, J. E., Ziomek, M. M., & Kowalchuk, R. K. (2010). Assessing relational learning deficits in perspective-taking in children with high-functioning autism spectrum disorder. *The Psychological Record, 57*(1), 4.

Roux, A. M., Shattuck, P. T., Rast, J. E., Rava, J. A., & Anderson, K. A. (2015*). National autism indicators report: Transition into young adulthood.* Philadelphia, PA: Life Course Outcomes Research Program, A. J. Drexel Autism Institute, Drexel University.

Scherf, K. S., Luna, B., Kimchi, R., Minshew, N., & Behrmann, M. (2009). Emergence of global shape processing continues through adolescence. *Child Development, 80*(1), 162-177.

Sofronoff, K., Dark, E., & Stone, V. (2011). Social vulnerability and bullying in children with Asperger syndrome. *Autism, 15*(3), 355-372.

Soulières, I., Mottron, L., Saumier, D., & Larochelle, S. (2007). Atypical categorical perception in autism: Autonomy of discrimination?. *Journal of Autism and Developmental Disorders, 37*(3), 481-490.

Stichter, J. P., Herzog, M. J., Visovsky, K., Schmidt, C., Randolph, J., Schultz, T., & Gage, N. (2010). Social competence intervention for youth with Asperger syndrome and high-functioning autism: An initial investigation. *Journal of Autism and Developmental Disorders, 40*(9), 1067-1079.

Stribling, P., Rae, J., & Dickerson, P. (2009). Using conversation analysis to explore the recurrence of a topic in the talk of a boy with an autism spectrum disorder. *Clinical Linguistics & Phonetics, 23*(8), 555-582.

Tanidir, C., & Mukaddes, N. M. (2014). Referral pattern and special interests in children and adolescents with Asperger syndrome: A Turkish referred sample. *Autism, 18*(2), 178-184.

Vermeulen, P. (2012). *Autism as context blindness.* Shawnee Mission, KS: AAPC Publishing.

Volkmar, F., Siegel, M., Woodbury-Smith, M., King, B., McCracken, J., & State, M. (2014). Practice parameter for the assessment and treatment of children and adolescents with autism spectrum disorder. *Journal of the American Academy of Child & Adolescent Psychiatry, 53*(2), 237-257.

Wang, P., & Spillane, A. (2009). Evidence-based social skills interventions for children with autism: A meta-analysis. *Education and Training in Developmental Disabilities,* 318-342.

White, S. W., Koenig, K., & Scahill, L. (2007). Social skills development in children with autism spectrum disorders: A review of the intervention research. *Journal of Autism and Developmental Disorders, 37*(10), 1858-1868.

Williams, D. L., Cherkassky, V. L., Mason, R. A., Keller, T. A., Minshew, N. J., & Just, M. A. (2013), Brain function differences in language processing in children and adults with autism. *Autism Research, 6*(4), 288-302. doi:10.1002/aur.1291

Williams, D. L., Goldstein, G., & Minshew, N. J. (2006). The profile of memory function in children with autism. *Neuropsychology, 20*(1), 21.

Wilson, C. E., Brock, J., & Palermo, R. (2010). Attention to social stimuli and facial identity recognition skills in autism spectrum disorder. *Journal of Intellectual Disability Research, 54*(12), 1104-1115.

Wing, K. (1981). Asperger's syndrome: A clinical account. *Psychological Medicine, 11*, 115-129.

APPENDICES

- A. Letter to Parent(s)
- B. Conversation Framework
- C. Conversation Topics List
- D. Conversation Topics List (With Pictures for Nonreaders)
- E. Topic
- F. General vs. Specific
- G. Weight
- H. Emotion List
- I. Timing
- J. Conversation vs. Whole-Group Listening
- K. Main Topic of Conversation
- L. Carrier Phrases for Asking Questions
- M. Carrier Phrases for Telling Stories
- N. Scripts for Comments
- O. Questions, Stories, Comments Cheat Sheet 1
- P. Questions, Stories, Comments Cheat Sheet 2
- Q. Bridge Visual
- R. Common Category Chart
- S. Transition Cards
- T. Data Collection Sheet Q S C
- U. Data Collection Sheet Bridging Topics
- V. Data Collection Sheet Self Report
- W. Guidelines for Balancing Conversation With Different Types of Participants
- X. Assessment for Balancing Questions, Stories, and Comments – Tally Mark Chart

APPENDIX A

Letter Parent(s)

Dear Parents,

We look forward to partnering with you to serve your child in the area of conversation skills. We will be using the Conversation Framework, which is a step-by-step, evidence-based practice for teaching conversation to high-functioning individuals with an autism spectrum disorder (HF-ASD) and related disabilities.

There are many indications that a person has a deficit in conversation, including his or her brain "going blank," telling long-winded stories, giving too much detail in stories with less regard to the main point, remaining quiet or giving short responses in conversation, preference for conversation with someone not one's own age, feeling interrupted often, and interrupting others. Because conversation deficits are so varied, conversation groups have to be individualized to the needs of each participant to maximize the speed at which each student learns. For example, if a student who asks numerous questions is paired with somebody who tells long-winded stories, it is possible for the student who carries on with numerous questions will reinforce the other person's stories in a negative way. With this in mind, conversational strengths *and* needs will be considered when creating a conversation group or adding a new student to an existing group. Other things that we will consider include age, interests, and gender.

The Conversation Framework provides a three-step framework, including (a) identifying the topic; (b) balancing asking questions, telling stories, and making comments within 0-2 seconds; and (c) bridging the topic. These steps are equally important but are taught in sequential order starting with identifying the topic. Once a step has been mastered across environments, your child will be ready to move onto the next step. It is important that too much is not taught at one time, which is why the focus is on one step at a time.

Your child is working on the following step of the Conversation Framework:

> ___ **Step 1 – Identify the Topic**
> Knowing the topic is the first step toward having an effective conversation. The concept of "on topic" vs. "off topic" is addressed during this step. Identifying the Topic is first because it is required to make on-topic contributions and bridge the topic, which are the next steps.
>
> ___ **Step 2 – Balance Asking Questions, Telling Stories, and Making Comments Within 0-2 Seconds**
> The term *balance* is used here to refer to creating an equal distribution of questions, stories, and comments both with regard to one's own utterances and in proportion to others' statements. This is second because the student must be able to contribute to the conversation and keep one topic going well before needing to switch to a different topic. This allows the student to find out about the topic at hand.
>
> ___ **Balance Asking Questions Within 0-2 Seconds**
> Asking questions is essential to keeping a conversation going. Asking questions allows you to find out information from others, as well as let someone know you are interested in what they have to say. There are times we may not be interested in what someone has to say, but we ask a question anyway because it shows interest in others.

APPENDICES

> ___ **BalanceTelling Stories Within 0-2 Seconds**
> Telling stories is a significant component of having a conversation. Conversations without stories are boring. Stories allow you to give information in a logical format. They are important because they allow others to get to know you and entertain people.
>
> ___ **Balance Making Comments Within 0-2 Seconds**
> Making relevant comments is an important part of mastering conversation. Making comments allows you to show interest in what others are saying and makes others feel comfortable.
>
> ___ **Step 3 – Bridge the Topic**
> Bridging the topic is a vital skill for maintaining a longer conversation. Once the other areas of the Conversation Framework are mastered, the last step is learning to bridge from one topic to a related topic without appearing to make a drastic change in the conversation.

Because we will remain on this step until mastery during our sessions, I will not send home detailed notes each week unless they are requested or required as part of your child's IEP. The Conversation Framework has been in use since 2005 and has helped hundreds of students overcome the anxiety of conversation and address their specific deficits. We hope your child will find the same success.

Please do not hesitate to contact me with any questions pertaining to your child.

Sincerely,

APPENDIX B

Conversation Framework

STEP 1: Identify the Topic
Topic _____
STEP 2: Balance Asking Questions, Telling Stories, and Making Comments Within 0-2 Seconds
Q Asking Questions
S Telling Stories
C Making Comments
STEP 3: Bridge the Topic

APPENDIX C

Conversation Topics List

CONVERSATION TOPICS	
• People & Lives	• Books
• School	• Places
• Job	• Sports
• Hobbies & Interests	• Food
• Current Events	• Weather
• News	• Holidays
• Weekend	• Vacations
• TV Shows	• Family & Pets
• Movies	• Where You Are (right now)
• Music	• Who Is With You (right now)
• Electronics	• Weird Things

APPENDIX D

Conversation Topics List (With Pictures for Nonreaders)

CONVERSATION TOPICS		
• People & Lives	• Movies	• Weather
• School	• Music	• Holidays
• Job	• Electronics	• Vacations
• Hobbies & Interests	• Books	• Family & Pets
• Current Events	• Places	• Where You Are (right now)
• News	• Sports	• Who Is With You (right now)
• Weekend	• Food	• Weird Things
• TV Shows		

APPENDIX E
TOPIC

THE TOPIC IS WHAT THE WHOLE THING IS ABOUT.

THE TOPIC IS WHAT THE PERSON IS TALKING ABOUT.

A TOPIC IS THE MAIN POINT OF WHAT IS BEING SAID.

APPENDIX F
GENERAL vs. SPECIFIC

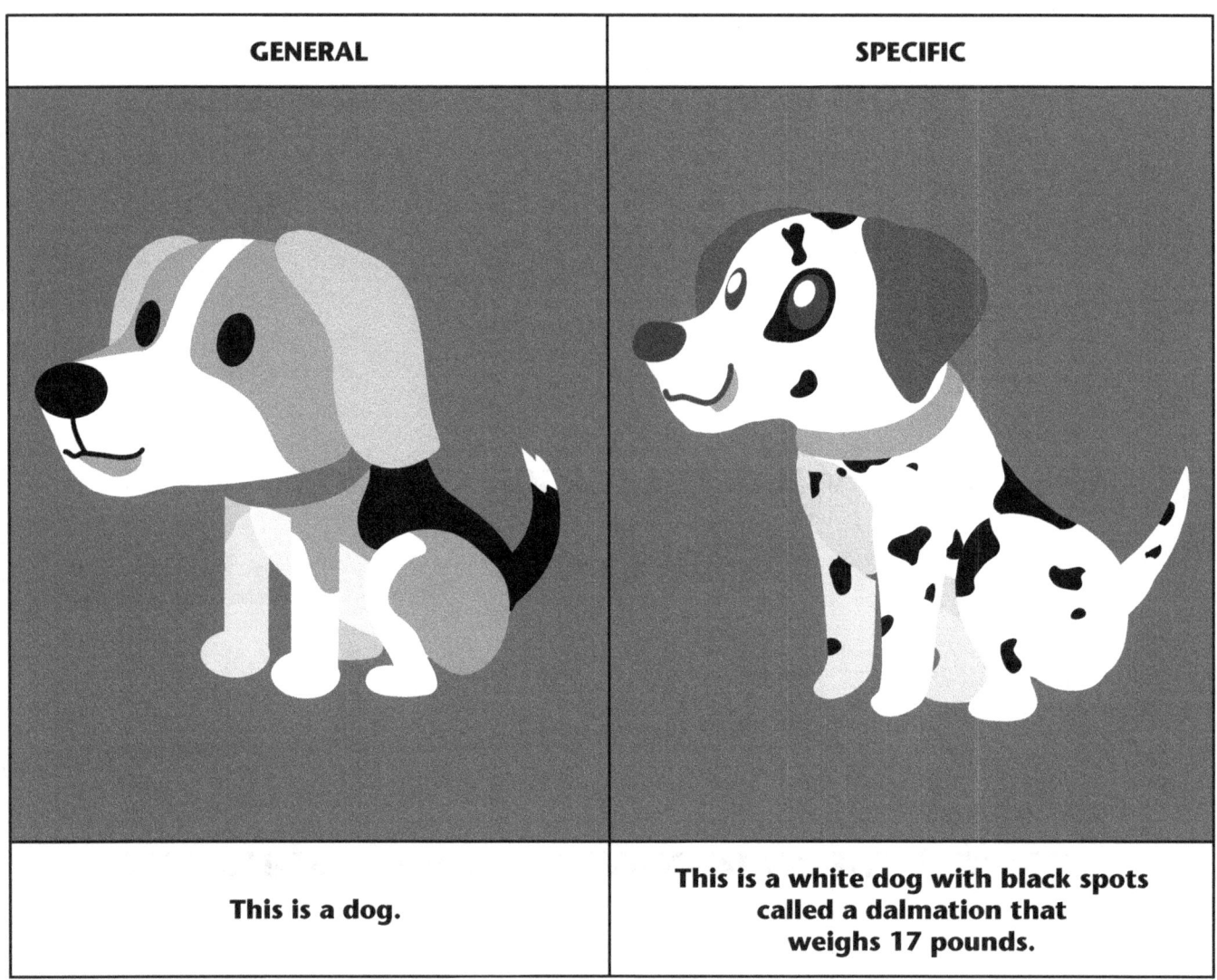

APPENDIX G

Weight

Light	**Medium**	**Heavy**
(joking)	**(neutral)**	**(serious)**

| **Joking** | | **Serious** |

APPENDIX H

Basic Emotion List

	Afraid
	Angry
	Annoyed
	Anxious
	Awkward
	Bored
	Calm
	Confident
	Confused
	Disappointed
	Disgusted
	Doubt
	Embarrassed
	Excited
	Frustrated
	Guilty
	Happy
	Hopeful

	Hyper
	Impatient
	Interested
	Irritated
	Jealous
	Lonely
	Loved
	Mischievous
	Nervous
	Overwhelmed
	Pain
	Panicked
	Patient
	Peace
	Proud
	Relaxed
	Sad
	Sarcastic

	Scared
	Shocked (bad)
	Shocked (good)
	Shy
	Silly
	Skeptical
	Sneaky
	Sorry
	Stressed
	Surprised (bad)
	Surprised (good)
	Suspicious
	Tired
	Uncomfortable
	Uninterested
	Unloved
	Upset
	Worried

APPENDIX H

Advanced Emotion List

	Afraid
	Angry
	Annoyed
	Anxious
	Ashamed
	Awkward
	Bashful
	Betrayed
	Bored
	Brave
	Calm
	Caring
	Concerned
	Confident
	Confused
	Content
	Defensive
	Disappointed
	Disbelief
	Disgusted
	Doubt
	Embarrassed
	Excited
	Excluded
	Exhausted

	Flirtatious
	Frustrated
	Guilty
	Happy
	Hesitant
	Hopeful
	Hopeless
	Hurt
	Hyper
	Impatient
	Interested
	Irritated
	Jealous
	Lonely
	Loved
	Mischievous
	Nervous
	Overwhelmed
	Pain
	Panicked
	Patient
	Peace
	Proud
	Relaxed
	Remorseful

	Sad
	Sarcastic
	Scared
	Shocked (bad)
	Shocked (good)
	Shy
	Silly
	Skeptical
	Smug
	Sneaky
	Sorry
	Stressed
	Surprised (bad)
	Surprised (good)
	Suspicious
	Tense
	Tired
	Uncomfortable
	Understanding
	Unimpressed
	Uninterested
	Unloved
	Unsure
	Upset
	Worried

APPENDIX I

TIMING

> # Timing

APPENDICES

APPENDIX J

Conversation vs. Whole-Group Listening

Is It ...

1. Conversation

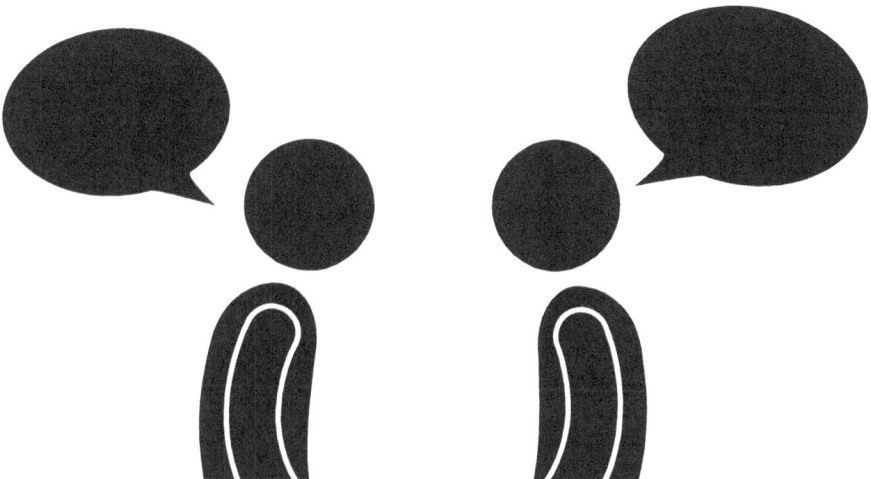

OR

2. Whole-Group Listening

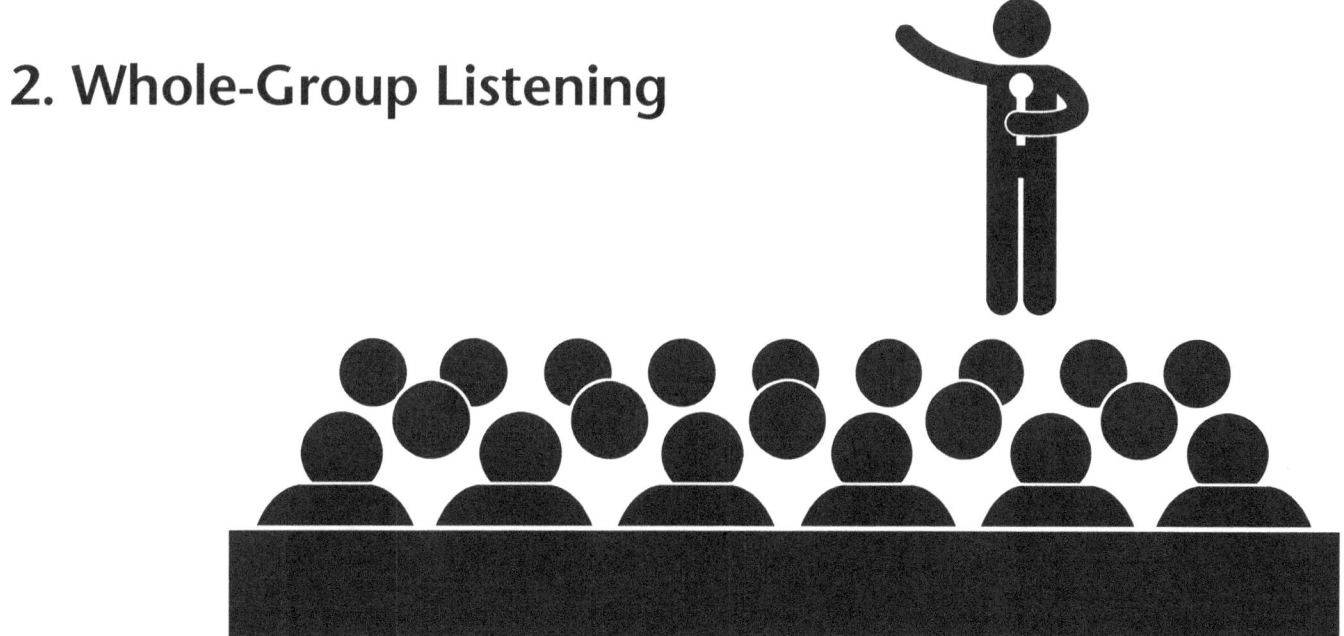

APPENDIX K

Main Topic of Conversation

1. **Asking Questions**

2. **Making Comments**

3. **Telling Stories**

The main topic is _____.

Ask one question to start a conversation and two follow-up questions on topic!

APPENDIX L

Carrier Phrases for Asking Questions

Asking Questions

Who ___?

What ___?

When ___?

Where ___?

Why ___?

How ___?

Do you ___?

Have you ___?

APPENDIX M

Carrier Phrases for Telling Stories

Telling Stories

I _____.

One time _____.

Once _____.

APPENDIX N

Scripts for Comments

Positive

Cool.

Me, too.

I want to go.

That's awesome.

Negative

That's awful.

I'm sorry to hear that.

APPENDIX O

Questions, Stories, Comments, Cheat Sheet 1

Asking Questions

Who __?	Have you ___?
What __?	How ___?
When __?	Where ___?
Do you ___?	What else ___?

Telling Stories

One time …

I …

Once …

Making Comments

Cool.

Me, too.

I haven't seen it.

APPENDIX P

Questions, Stories, Comments, Cheat Sheet 2

Conversation

New People

Name
Grade
Hobbies/Interests
Where They Live
Where You Are
Who You Are With
Scan & Ask Question

At least 90% of conversation with new people is asking questions.

Three Parts of Conversation

1. Asking Questions
2. Telling Stories
3. Making Comments

General Conversation Topics

People & Lives
School
Job
Hobbies & Interests
Current Events
News
Weekend
TV Shows
Movies
Music
Electronics
Books
Places
Sports
Food
Weather
Holidays
Vacations
Family & Pets
Where You Are (right now)
Who Is With You (right now)
Weird Things

Asking Questions

Have you heard _____?
Did you see _____?
What _____?

Telling Stories

One time . . .
I . . .
Once . . .

Making Comments

Cool.
Me too.
That's awesome.
That's awful.
I'm sorry to hear that.

Bridging Topics

Speaking of . . .
This reminds me of . . .

Making Connections with Friends

I heard . . .
Remember when . . .

APPENDIX Q

Bridge Visual

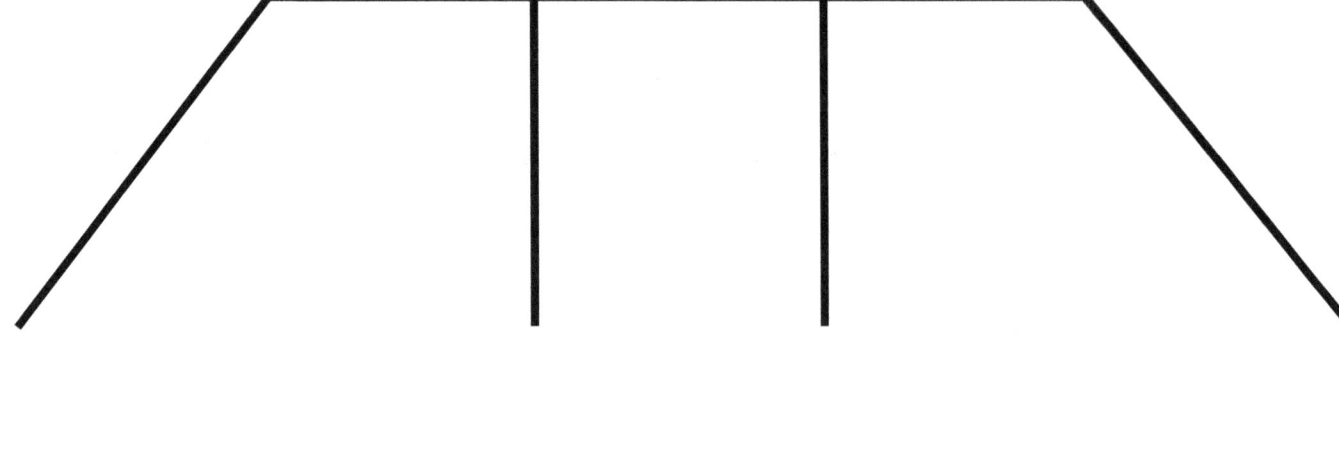

Speaking of ... _____

That reminds me of ... _____

APPENDIX Q

Bridge Topics

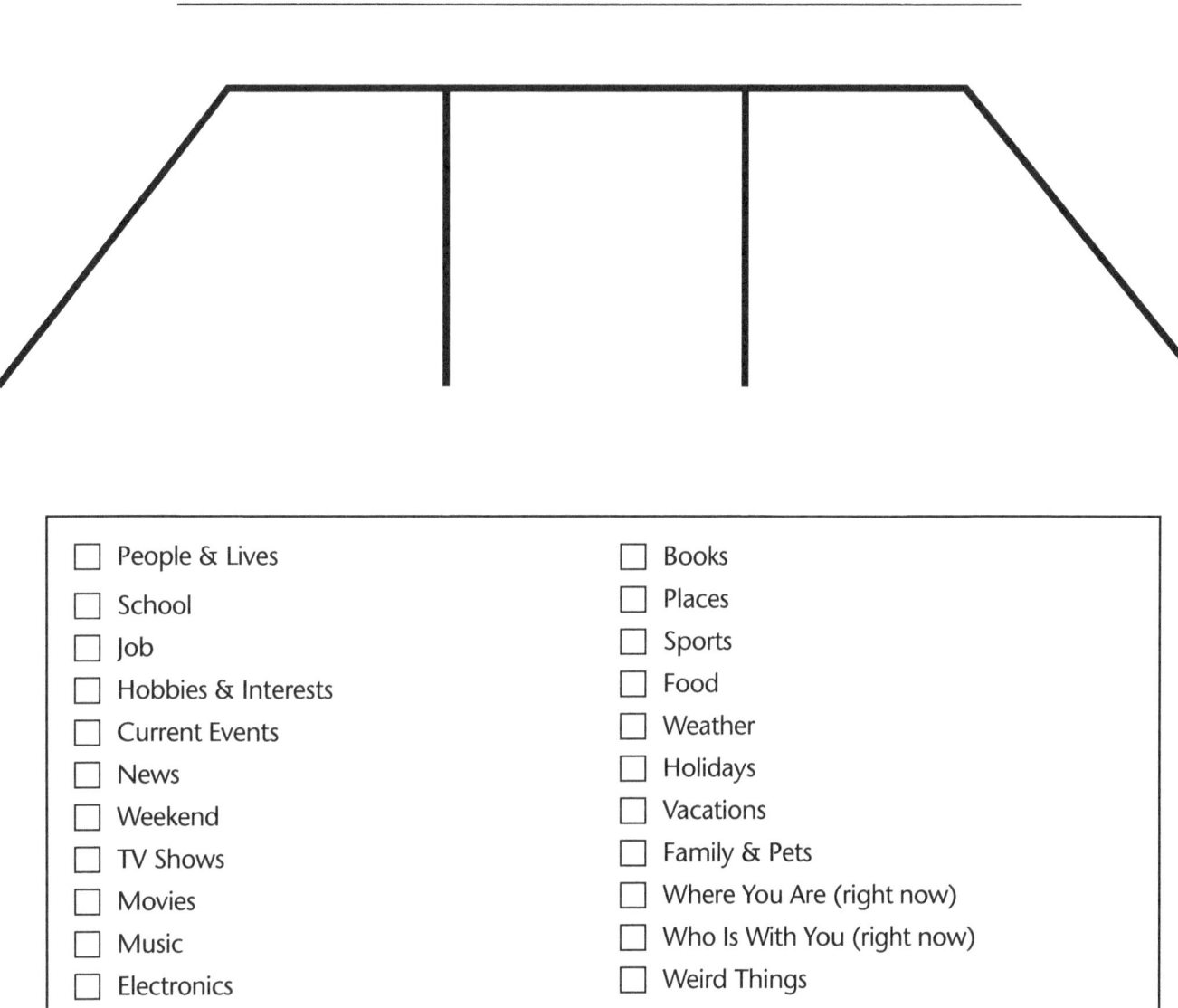

- ☐ People & Lives
- ☐ School
- ☐ Job
- ☐ Hobbies & Interests
- ☐ Current Events
- ☐ News
- ☐ Weekend
- ☐ TV Shows
- ☐ Movies
- ☐ Music
- ☐ Electronics
- ☐ Books
- ☐ Places
- ☐ Sports
- ☐ Food
- ☐ Weather
- ☐ Holidays
- ☐ Vacations
- ☐ Family & Pets
- ☐ Where You Are (right now)
- ☐ Who Is With You (right now)
- ☐ Weird Things

APPENDIX R

Common Category Chart

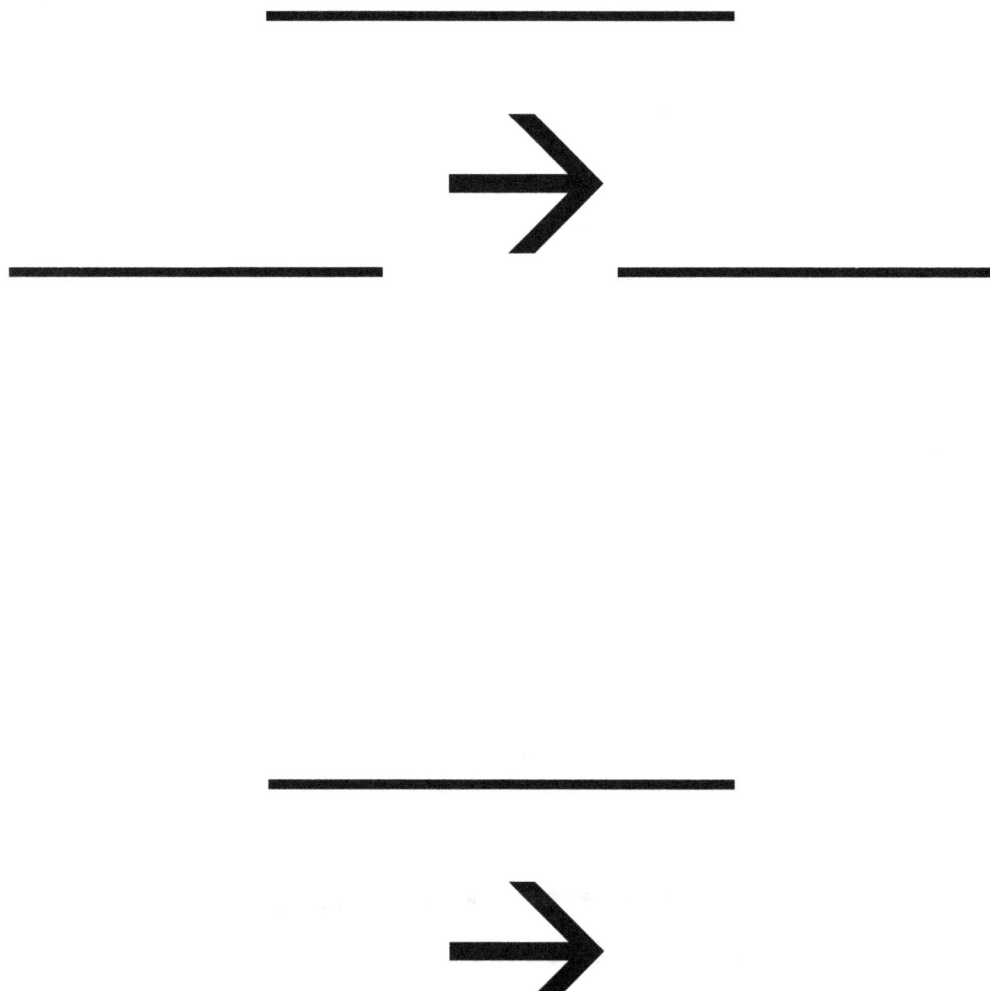

184

APPENDICES

APPENDIX S

Transition Cards

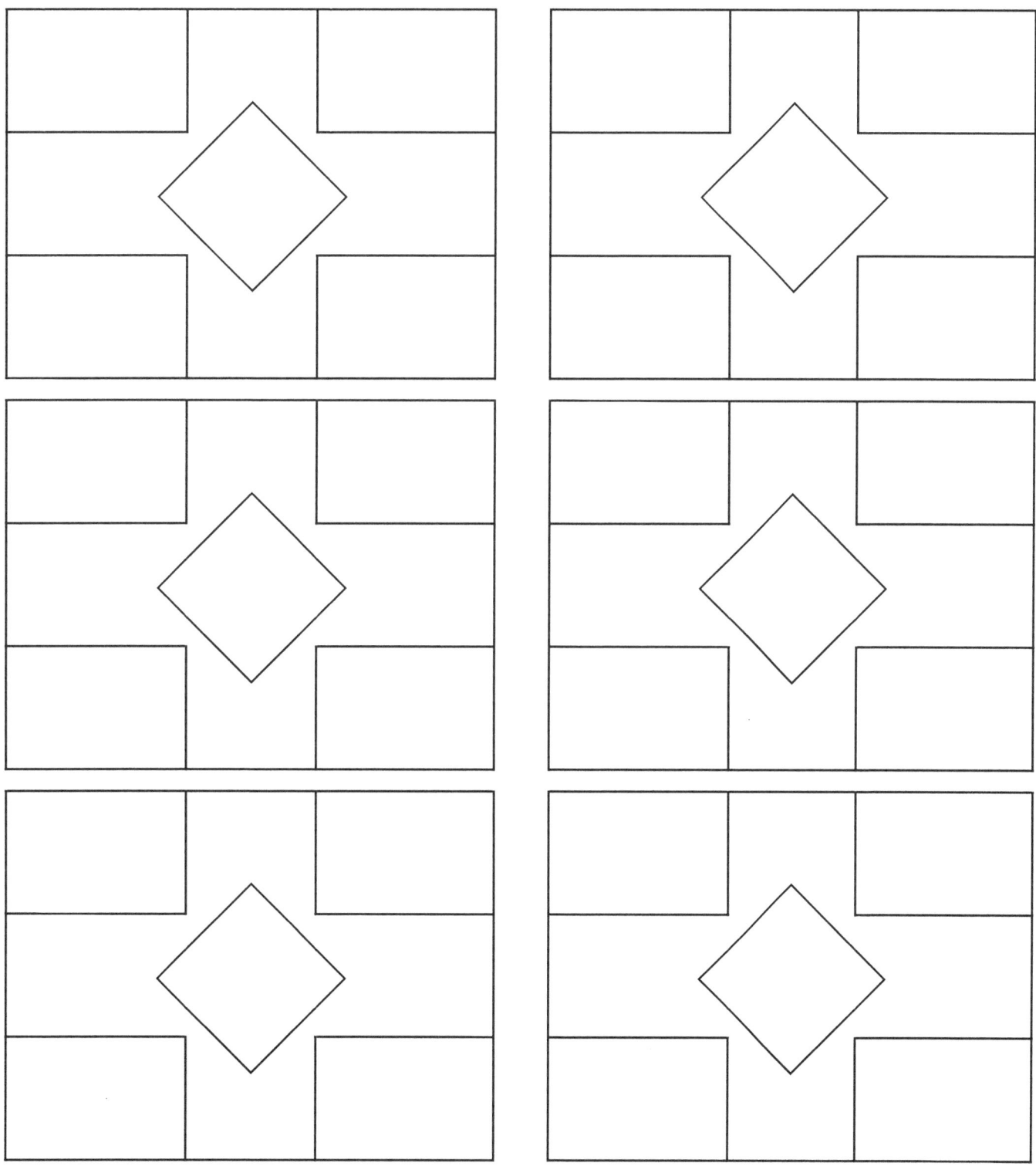

185

TALK WITH ME

APPENDIX S

General/Specific Transition Cards

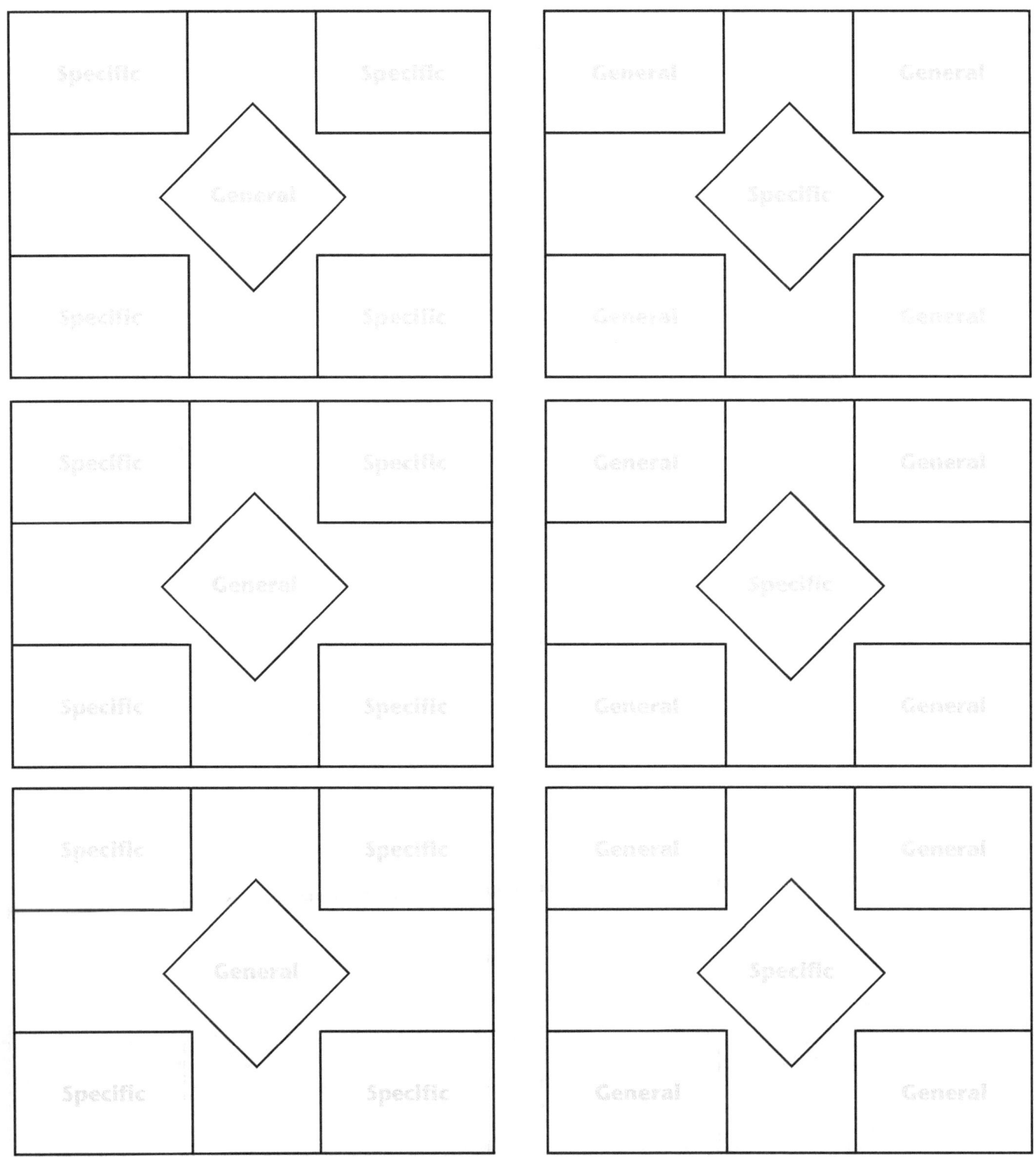

186

APPENDIX T

Data Collection Sheet, Q S C

Student Name _____ Grade _____ Evaluator _____

Directions: For each topic, use a tally mark to represent each question, story, and comment. This data collection is for tracking one student.

Topic _____

Date	Questions	Stories	Comments

Topic _____

Date	Questions	Stories	Comments

Topic _____

Date	Questions	Stories	Comments

Topic _____

Date	Questions	Stories	Comments

APPENDIX U
Data Collection Sheet, Bridging Topics

Conversation Skills

Date: _____ Setting: _____ Initials: _____

Directions: Make a tally mark only when student engages in independent components of conversation.

	Asking Questions	Telling Stories	Making Comments	Bridging Topics (speaking of… that reminds me of..)
Name:* _____				
Name: _____				
Name: _____				

Topics: _____ → _____ → _____ → _____

_____ Student dominated the conversation
_____ Student had reciprocal conversation (back and forth; balanced)
_____ Student picked up on cues that friend was not interested in topic ____ N/O
_____ Student did not pick up on cues that friend was not interested in topic

Conversation Skills

Date: _____ Setting: _____ Initials: _____

Directions: Make a tally mark only when student engages in independent components of conversation.

	Asking Questions	Telling Stories	Making Comments	Bridging Topics (speaking of… that reminds me of..)
Name:* _____				
Name: _____				
Name: _____				

Topics: _____ → _____ → _____ → _____

_____ Student dominated the conversation
_____ Student had reciprocal conversation (back and forth; balanced)
_____ Student picked up on cues that friend was not interested in topic ____ N/O
_____ Student did not pick up on cues that friend was not interested in topic

APPENDIX V

Data Collection Sheet, Self-Report

Topics _____

Did I:

Ask question to start conversation/

☐ ☐

Ask follow-up questions/

☐ ☐ ☐

Tell related stories? (Ex: One time ..., I ...)

☐ ☐ ☐

Make comments to show interest? (ex: Cool, me too)

☐ ☐ ☐

OVERALL RATING:

☐ ☐ ☐

Excellent   **Okay**   **HELP!**

APPENDIX W

Guidelines for Balancing Conversation With Different Types of Participants

Balancing Conversation With Different Types of Participants

There are many types of individuals with HF-ASD who may be interested in participating in a conversation group setting. Common types include the following.

Monologuer

A "Monologuer" is someone who tells numerous stories or tells very long stories without asking any questions. Monologuers sometimes make comments but very rarely ask questions about others. At first glance, the conversation may look pretty balanced, but all of the Monologuer's stories tend to be extremely long, so no one else gets a chance to talk. If you tracked the conversation of a "Monologuer," it might look like this:

	Asking Questions	Telling Stories	Making Comments
Person 1	-	⤤ I	III

Refrain from putting a "Monologuer" in a conversation group with types to be discussed later such as "The Silent One" or a "Slow Responder." Groups with Monologuers must be carefully managed so all group members get something out of the group.

Interrogator

An interrogator is someone who only asks question with very few or no comments or stories. The conversation of an "Interrogator" may look like this:

	Asking Questions	Telling Stories	Making Comments
Person 1	⤤ ⤤	-	-

Be mindful of who you are placing with an "Interrogator" because the excessive questions can cause other participants to look like "Monologuers." Groups with interrogators must be very carefully managed.

Commenter

The "Commenter" is someone who makes short comments without asking questions or telling stories. This may be a result of (a) not paying attention to the conversation, (b) not knowing how to ask questions or tell stories, (c) knowing that one is supposed to contribute to the conversation but not feeling completely comfortable yet, or (d) copying something that someone else said in the conversation. The conversation of a "Commenter" may look like this:

	Asking Questions	Telling Stories	Making Comments
Person 1	-	-	⤤ ⤤

Refrain from putting a "Commenter" in a conversation group with a "Monologuer" unless you are able to balance conversation through support and direct instruction. Be sure to provide direct instruction on how to ask questions and tell stories in the context of a natural conversation.

APPENDICES

Slow Responder

The "Slow Responder" is someone who complains about not knowing what people are talking about, which may be due to the pace of the conversation or use of slang, inferences, inside jokes, etc. Students who are "Slow Responders" do not say much. When asked why, they typically respond that they did not know what everyone was talking about, others were talking too fast, or something similar. If allowed to have unlimited time to respond, a "Slow Responder" often takes more than 20 seconds to come up with a question, story, or comment. If you tracked the conversation of a "Slow Responder," it might look like this because she is not able to create the timing to contribute to the conversation:

	Asking Questions	**Telling Stories**	**Making Comments**
Person 1	-	-	-

Refrain from putting a "Slow Responder" in a conversation group with a "Monologuer" until "The Slow Responder" can contribute to a conversation within 0-2 seconds or support and direct instruction can make the conversation balanced.

The Silent One

"The Silent One" is someone who is able to ask good questions, tell good stories, and make good comments but does not feel comfortable speaking up in conversation using questions, stories, or comments. His hesitation time is typically extended, sometimes 60 seconds or longer – a much longer delay than that of the Slow Responder. If you tracked the conversation of "The Silent One," it might look like this:

	Asking Questions	**Telling Stories**	**Making Comments**
Person 1	-	-	-

Refrain from putting "The Silent One" in a conversation group with a "Monologuer" until "The Silent One" can contribute to a conversation within 0-2 seconds.

"Disinteres-Ted"

A conversation partner described as "Disinteres-Ted" often states, "I'm not interested in that" and does not engage if the conversation is not interesting to him. This is easily confused with a "Focuser." "Disinteres-Ted" talk about many different things, but if they are not interested in the current topic, they will say that they aren't interested or will not say anything at all. The conversation of the "Disinteres-Ted" may look like this:

	Asking Questions	**Telling Stories**	**Making Comments**
Person 1	-	IIII	I

Robot

The "Robot" is someone who uses memorized scripts during a conversation and whose conversation, as a result, sounds rehearsed. She may be fine in the beginning of the conversation because small talk typically follows a script, but she may have difficulty in any other conversation because she has memorized scripts for conversation without learning how to follow the flow of a conversation. This person is often monotone. The conversation can be balanced, but it often lacks connection.

Randomizer

Someone who is a "Randomizer" randomly talks about whatever is on his mind regardless of the topic of conversation. He switches to his topic of interest or something that captures his thought at the moment. This person is not recognizable from the Tally Mark Chart because he may be proficient at any part of conversation; however, he often tells more stories than comments or questions.

Renegade

A "Renegade" is someone who asks questions, tells stories, or makes comments in a strange or bizarre manner that does not fit the situation. For example, the "Renegade" may ask very specific questions such as the following:

> Mrs. Kerry: "I went to the zoo last week with my kids."
>
> Pause
>
> Mrs. Kerry: "What can you ask me about my trip to the zoo?"
>
> Renegade: "Did you see Ms. Lee at the zoo?"

In the above conversation, the Renegade knew that she was supposed to ask a question, but the question she came up with was too specific. This person is not recognizable from the Tally Mark Chart because she shows no specific deficit or strength in balancing asking questions, telling stories, or making comments. This person struggles with the content of the questions, stories, and comments.

Focuser

The "Focuser" appears to be so fixated or interested on a specific topic that he attempts to change every conversation to that subject. This is harder to recognize because there is no chart pattern that can depict it. This person may also be confused with "Disinteres-Ted." The difference is that the "Focuser" talks about the same thing almost every time you see her. She typically starts a conversation with a story or question about her topic of interest. She may ask questions that redirect the conversation to their topic of interest such as:

> Mrs. Kerry: "I went to the OCALICON conference in Ohio last week. It was pretty fun. I hung out with a lot of old friends."
>
> Focuser: "What interstates did you drive on when you were there?"

In the above conversation, the "Focuser" is fascinated with interstate highways, so he asks very specific questions about this topic on a frequent basis.

	Asking Questions	Telling Stories	Making Comments
Person 1	-	IIII	III

Story Topper

The "Story Topper" is someone who is constantly telling a story that is grander than the story before. This person is also known as a "One0Upper."

	Asking Questions	Telling Stories	Making Comments
Person 1	-	IIII	-

APPENDICES

APPENDIX X

Assessment for Balancing Questions, Stories, and Comments – Tally Mark Chart

Three People Date: _____

Directions: Write the names or initials of each student by the numbers to identify each person's individual performance. As the conversation begins, immediately begin tracking the conversation by making a tally mark to track each question, story, and comment.

Student's Name	Questions	Stories	Comments
1.			
2.			
3.			

Four People Date: _____

Directions: Write the names or initials of each student by the numbers to identify each person's individual performance. As the conversation begins, immediately begin tracking the conversation by making a tally mark to track each question, story, and comment.

Student's Name	Questions	Stories	Comments
1.			
2.			
3.			
4.			

Five People Date: _____

Directions: Write the names or initials of each student by the numbers to identify each person's individual performance. As the conversation begins, immediately begin tracking the conversation by making a tally mark to track each question, story, and comment.

Student's Name	Questions	Stories	Comments
1.			
2.			
3.			
4.			
5.			

Six People Date: _____

Directions: Write the names or initials of each student by the numbers to identify each person's individual performance. As the conversation begins, immediately begin tracking the conversation by making a tally mark to track each question, story, and comment.

Student's Name	Questions	Stories	Comments
1.			
2.			
3.			
4.			
5.			
6.			

Seven People

Directions: Write the names or initials of each student by the numbers to identify each person's individual performance. As the conversation begins, immediately begin tracking the conversation by making a tally mark to track each question, story, and comment.

Student's Name	Questions	Stories	Comments
1.			
2.			
3.			
4.			
5.			
6.			
7.			

Eight People

Directions: Write the names or initials of each student by the numbers to identify each person's individual performance. As the conversation begins, immediately begin tracking the conversation by making a tally mark to track each question, story, and comment.

Student's Name	Questions	Stories	Comments
1.			
2.			
3.			
4.			
5.			
6.			
7.			
8.			

Did you like this book?

Rate it and share your opinion!

BARNES & NOBLE
BOOKSELLERS
www.bn.com

amazon.com

Not what you expected? Tell us!

Most negative reviews occur when the book did not reach expectation. Did the description build any expectations that were not met? Let us know how we can do better.

Please drop us a line at info@fhautism.com.
Thank you so much for your support!

FUTURE HORIZONS

www.ingramcontent.com/pod-product-compliance
Lightning Source LLC
Chambersburg PA
CBHW081347080526
44588CB00016B/2406